MULTIPLE CHOICE QUESTIONS IN
CLINICAL EXAMINATION

Nicholas J Talley

MD (NSW), PhD (Syd), FRACP, FRCP (Edin), FACP, FACG, FAFPHM

Professor of Medicine
Department of Medicine
The University of Sydney
Nepean Hospital
Sydney, Australia

Simon O'Connor

FRACP, DDU

Cardiologist
Cardiology Unit
Woden Valley Hospital
Canberra, Australia

b
**Blackwell
Science**

D0897458

© 1996 MacLennan & Petty Pty Limited
809 Botany Road, Rosebery, NSW 2018, Australia

First published 1996

Distributed in the United Kingdom and Europe by
Blackwell Science Ltd
Osney Mead, Oxford OX2 OEL
Orders should be addressed to:
Marston Book Services Ltd
PO Box 269, Abingdon
Oxon OX14 4YN
Tel: +44 1235 465500
Fax: +44 1235 465555

A catalogue record for this title is available from the
British Library and the Library of Congress

ISBN: 0-632-04153-6

Printed and bound in Australia

PREFACE

*If you want to get out of medicine the fullest enjoyment,
be students all your lives.*

David Reisman (1867–1940)

What we have to learn to do, we learn by doing.

Aristotle (384–322 BC)

It is essential that history taking and physical examination be learned at the
bedside; experience and practice are good teachers. However, a core of knowledge, which must be constantly revised and brought up to date, remains a
fundamental requirement if clinical medicine of the highest standard is to be
practised. The 3rd Edition of *Clinical Examination* has been written to provide a
modern, systematic and comprehensive guide to the evaluation of patients and
the interpretation of the clinical findings. We have designed this book of multiple
choice questions to accompany the 3rd Edition in order to assist students of
medicine retain the core information. The book is meant primarily as an aid to
revision, and is not meant to grade students. Single-answer, multiple-answer and
other formats have been used to assist with understanding and revision.

We have purposely varied the degree of difficulty of the questions because
this book is meant to be an educational tool. However, we have included detailed
answers to each question to improve understanding. We have also provided page
cross-references to the 3rd Edition of *Clinical Examination* to promote further
reading. In order to ensure their clarity and relevance, we tested the questions on
final year medical students in mock examinations, and then revised the questions
and answers as needed. We have also had the questions and answers reviewed by
senior registrars and consultants in various subspecialities.

The book is divided into chapters that contain questions linked to each
chapter of *Clinical Examination*. A final quiz has been included for revision
purposes.

We hope that this book will prove both useful and enjoyable.

Nicholas J Talley
Simon O'Connor
May, 1996

ACKNOWLEDGMENTS

This paper will no doubt be found interesting
by those who take an interest in it.

John Dalton (1766–1844)

We would like to thank the following specialists who helped us review, revise or develop the questions and answers in this book. We are very grateful for their help, but we of course take responsibility for the content.

Professor P Boyce	Dr D Currow	Dr P McManis
Dr D S Coulshed	Dr B Frankum	Dr S Nandurkar
Dr S J Coulshed	Dr T O'Meagan	Dr N A Talley

Despite our best efforts, factual errors may still have been included. If you have any questions or suggestions, please write to us care of the publisher.

CONTENTS

DIRECTIONS

Each of the questions in these chapters is followed by answers or by completions of a statement. Select each of the answers that you believe to be true. More than one answer may be correct unless it is specified that you should choose the one best answer.

Chapter 1

The General Principles of History Taking

Here am I dying of a hundred good symptoms.

Alexander Pope (1688–1744)

1-1 Questions about a patient's smoking habits are important because of the clinical associations. These associations include:

(a) carcinoma of the lung
(b) chronic liver disease
(c) peripheral vascular disease
(d) coronary artery disease
(e) diabetes mellitus.

1-2 Alcohol consumption must be asked about non-judgmentally because a more honest answer is likely to be obtained. Which of the following statements are true about alcohol?

(a) One glass of wine contains approximately 10g
(b) Alcohol consumption in men is considered safe to a level of 80g a day
(c) Men may safely consume more alcohol than women
(d) Cardiac arrhythmias may be precipitated by consumption of large amounts of alcohol
(e) Alcohol does not cause chronic liver disease.

Photograph 1.1

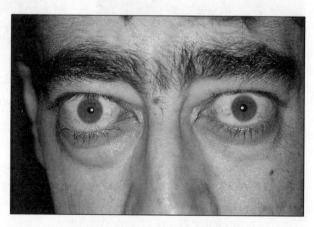

1-3 Apart from asking the patient in Photograph 1.1 about his eyes, which of the following features on history taking is likely to produce the most helpful information?

1

(a)   A history of constipation over many years
(b)   Recent intolerance of cold weather
(c)   Loss of weight despite a normal diet
(d)   Ankle swelling from oedema
(e)   Heavy smoking for many years.

1-4   As part of the general history-taking for women, a menstrual history should be obtained. This is important because:

(a)   Women of child-bearing age must be asked about the possibility of pregnancy
      because
(b)   it may be unsafe to use certain drugs and to perform radiological procedures in pregnant woman.

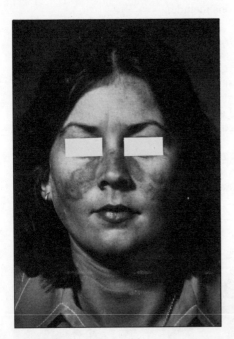

Photograph 1.2

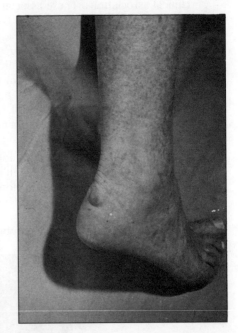

Photograph 1.3

1-5   The woman in Photograph 1.2 has presented with frontal hair loss. Important questions to ask her that might help with the diagnosis include:

(a)   duration of her facial rash
(b)   presence of any urinary symptoms
(c)   use of antihypertensive drugs
(d)   joint symptoms
(e)   smoking history.

1-6   The lump on this patient's Achilles tendon was an incidental finding and the patient was surprised when questions were asked about it. Which of the following aspects in subsequent history taking would be important?

(a)   a history of chronic liver disease
(b)   a history of smoking
(c)   a history of exertional chest pain
(d)   a family history of coronary artery disease
(e)   a history of arthritis.

1-7   When the patient in Photograph 1.3 is examined, similar lesions might be found:

(a)   on the extensor surfaces of the elbows
(b)   on the abdominal wall
(c)   on the eyelids
(d)   in the axillae
(e)   on the scalp.

1-8   When a man who needs urgent drug treatment for a life-threatening cardiac arrhythmia is questioned about allergies, he states: 'I am allergic to all drugs and chemical substances'. The most appropriate course of action in these circumstances is (choose the one best answer):

(a)   to ignore such foolishness
(b)   to use only drugs unlikely to cause allergies
(c)   to allow the arrhythmia to run its course
(d)   to attempt to find out what the exact manifestations of previous allergic reactions were, and what drugs were involved
(e)   to get the patient to give you permission for treatment at his own risk.

Chapter 2

The General Principles of Physical Examination

Either he's dead or my watch has stopped.

Groucho Marx (1895–1977)

2-1 The patient in Photograph 2.1:

   (a) should be examined from the other side of the bed
   (b) is in the correct position for the examination of the gastrointestinal system
   (c) is in the correct position for the examination of the cardiovascular system
   (d) is in the correct position for the examination of the cranial nerves
   (e) is probably not suffering from severe orthopnoea.

Photograph 2.1

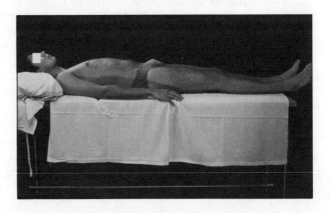

2-2 Which one of the following diagnoses cannot be made or strongly suspected on inspection alone (choose the one best answer)?

   (a) jaundice
   (b) obesity
   (c) female virilisation
   (d) Cushing's syndrome
   (e) cardiac failure.

Photograph 2.2

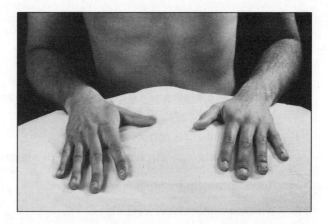

2-3 If a patient has joint or hand symptoms, formal inspection followed by examination of the hands is indicated. The hands should be placed as shown in Photograph 2.2. The following may all be noted on inspection alone EXCEPT (choose the one best answer):

(a) psoriatic nail changes
(b) tendon crepitus
(c) joint deformity
(d) palmar erythema
(e) acromegalic changes.

2-4 The most common cause of pallor as an incidental finding is:

(a) anaemia with a haemoglobin below 70g/L
(b) shock
(c) cold weather
(d) severe aortic stenosis
(e) less than average skin pigmentation.

2-5 Which statement is correct?

(a) When a patient who is anaemic is examined, the absence of cyanosis does not exclude hypoxia
because
(b) more than 50g/L of deoxygenated blood must be present for the skin to appear blue.

2-6 Peripheral cyanosis may be noted in patients with suspected cardiovascular or respiratory disease. Which of the following are true about peripheral cyanosis?

(a) It does not affect the tongue.
(b) It occurs when the tissues extract more oxygen than normal from the blood.
(c) It is a reliable sign of disease.
(d) It may indicate arterial occlusion.
(e) It is always present when the patient has central cyanosis.

2-7   Pallor is often best appreciated by standing back from the patient and undertaking a careful general inspection. Pallor:

(a)   may be a sign of anaemia
(b)   may be normal in certain people
(c)   is usually present in the presence of reduced cardiac output and shock
(d)   is more significant if it involves the skin creases
(e)   is a reliable sign of anaemia.

2-8   Which statement is correct?

(a)   Cyanosis occurs in some patients with congenital heart disease
      because
(b)   left-to-right shunting of blood occurs.

2-9   Which statement is correct?

(a)   Central cyanosis is not always due to hypoxia
      because
(b)   it may occur in some rare haemoglobin abnormalities.

2-10   The clinical term 'shock' has a rather different meaning from that in common use. Causes of medically defined shock include:

(a)   coming across a completely unexpected question in the final examination
(b)   myocardial infarction
(c)   anaphylaxis
(d)   angina
(e)   Gram-negative sepsis.

2-11   Inspection of a patient's fingernails can be rewarding for the clinician. Which of the following may be suspected from such an examination?

(a)   Cigarette smoking
(b)   Infective endocarditis
(c)   Carcinoma of the pancreas
(d)   Thyrotoxicosis
(e)   Diabetes insipidus.

Chapter 3

The Cardiovascular System

A man is as old as his arteries.

Thomas Sydenham

3-1 The patient in Photograph 3.1

(a) is incorrectly placed for the cardiovascular examination
because
(b) the height of jugular venous pulse (JVP) is best assessed when the patient is lying flat.

Photograph 3.1

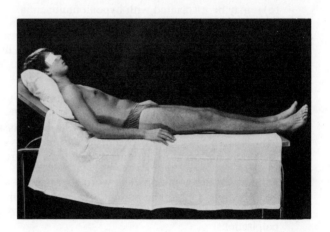

3-2 A diagnosis of coronary artery disease may often be strongly suspected simply on the basis of the history. A patient who has severe coronary artery disease:

(a) will always have angina
(b) will often describe a feeling of chest tightness occurring with exertion
(c) may admit to chest discomfort or tightness but deny any pain
(d) will always have a history of previous angina if questioned at the time a myocardial infarct has occurred
(e) may experience only dyspnoea on exertion.

3-3 The history can provide information about the probable severity of a patient's coronary artery disease. A patient with angina:

(a)   who has Class 4 symptoms only experiences symptoms during intense activity

(b)   may describe a feeling of discomfort in the throat associated with exertion but no abnormality involving the chest itself

(c)   is considered unstable if the symptoms have only recently begun

(d)   is considered stable when episodes occur at rest

(e)   will usually have symptoms relieved rapidly by sublingual nitrates.

3-4   A woman with chest tightness unrelated to exertion:

(a)   will almost certainly have coronary artery disease
because

(b)   other causes of chest pain are rare in women.

3-5   Ankle oedema is something patients may complain about; it can be a symptom or a sign. Sometimes only adipose tissue is the cause of the swelling. True ankle oedema:

(a)   is usually due to cardiac failure

(b)   tends to be worse later in the day

(c)   is often seen following the use of vasodilating drugs

(d)   may indicate deep venous thrombosis

(e)   may be associated with hypoalbuminaemia.

3-6   Dyspnoea means 'bad breathing' in Greek and is a common symptom. A patient may also appear dyspnoeic at rest or when undressing for the examination. This makes it a sign as well as a symptom. When dyspnoea is due to cardiac failure, it:

(a)   suggests that the aetiology is ischaemic heart disease

(b)   is often associated with orthopnoea

(c)   is a poor prognostic symptom following myocardial infarction

(d)   is often associated with a history of previous cardiac disease

(e)   does not occur in patients with valvular heart disease.

3-7   Palpitations are common. The word suggests the abnormal awareness of the heart beating. Unless the patient is seen during an attack, careful questioning is needed to help work out the likely diagnosis. A patient who complains of palpitations:

(a)   almost always has significant cardiac disease

(b)   is more likely to have an abnormal rhythm if the episodes are of sudden onset and offset than if they are gradual

(c)   may be able to terminate the episodes by performing the Valsalva manoeuvre if he or she is experiencing paroxysmal atrial fibrillation

(d)   probably has an abnormal rhythm if the heart rate is greater than 150 beats per minute at rest

(e)   may simply have an unexpected awareness of sinus rhythm.

3-8   The cardiac history must include questions about the important risk factors for coronary artery disease. This is because the presence of these risk factors (especially multiple factors) increases the likelihood that symptoms suggestive of ischaemic heart disease are indeed cardiac in origin. The following are risk factors for ischaemic heart disease:

* (a) smoking
  (b) coronary artery disease in second-degree relatives
* (c) a total serum cholesterol level above 5.2mmols/L
  (d) peptic ulceration
  (e) a difficult job.

3-9 Finger (and toe) clubbing are only rarely noticed by a patient but the trained clinician should notice them immediately on first examining a patient. Although its mechanism is not well understood, the causes of clubbing include:

  (a) carcinoma of the lung
  (b) infective endocarditis
  (c) thyrotoxicosis
  (d) a familial tendency
  (e) cyanotic congenital heart disease.

3-10 Atrial fibrillation is a common arrhythmia. It is increasingly common in old age. It sometimes occurs in medical students 12 to 14 hours after an alcoholic binge. Patients with atrial fibrillation:

  (a) are always aware of palpitations
  (b) always have a heart rate greater than 90 beats per minute
* (c) often have a ventricular rate of over 150 beats per minute if they are untreated
* (d) have an irregularly irregular pulse
  (e) always have serious underlying heart disease.

3-11 Measuring the blood pressure is an important part of the physical examination. To obtain an accurate reading certain aspects of the measurement must be understood (even though blood pressure can now be taken by machines which produce beeping noises and digital readouts). When the blood pressure is measured:

  (a) a 12.5cm cuff is suitable for all patients
  (b) the systolic blood pressure is determined by the appearance of the first Korotkoff sound
  (c) the diastolic blood pressure is said to occur at the point at which the Korotkoff sounds decrease suddenly
  (d) there may be no phase V in patients with aortic regurgitation
  (e) the systolic blood pressure may normally vary between the arms by up to 10mmHg.

3-12 Pulsations of the internal jugular vein can seem mysterious and complicated and patients may be surprised at the time clinicians spend staring at their necks. Pulsations of the internal jugular vein:

* (a) reflect movements of the top of a column of blood extending into the right atrium
  (b) are best measured with the patient lying flat
* (c) flicker twice with each cardiac cycle unless the patient is in atrial fibrillation
  (d) should normally rise on inspiration (Kussmaul's sign)
  (e) usually exhibit large v waves in a patient with mitral regurgitation.

3-13   Much can be learned about the heart before the stethoscope is applied to the praecordium. Time spent on careful assessment of the apex beat is rewarding. The apex beat:

    (a)   can normally be felt in the fifth intercostal space just to the left of the sternum

    (b)   may feel displaced in a patient with cardiac failure

    (c)   may have a tapping quality in patients with mitral regurgitation

    (d)   should always be palpable

    (e)   is normally felt over an area the size of a 20 cent piece.

Photograph 3.2

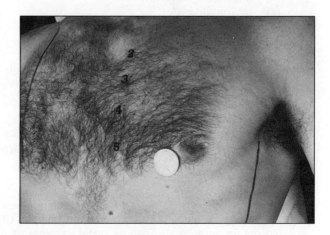

3-14   When the apex beat is not palpable in the position shown in Photograph 3.2, the most likely explanation is (choose the one best answer):

    (a)   dextrocardia

    (b)   cardiomegaly

    (c)   pericardial effusion

    (d)   severe mitral regurgitation

    (e)   a thick chest wall.

3-15   The first heart sound:

    (a)   has two components

        because

    (b)   it occurs during mitral and tricuspid valve closure.

3-16   The pulmonary component of the second heart sound (P2):

    (a)   is usually loud on inspiration

        because

    (b)   of increased venous return to the right ventricle.

3-17   When a patient presents with dyspnoea it is important to examine for signs of heart failure. A third heart sound represents an abnormality that:

(a)   is often described as causing a gallop rhythm
(b)   may be a normal variant in children and young adults
(c)   is a reliable sign of cardiac failure in adults
(d)   may be normal in pregnant women
(e)   is probably related to an increased rate or volume of ventricular filling.

3-18   A summation gallop:

(a)   usually occurs at heart rates greater than 120 beats per minute
        because
(b)   it is due to the superimposition of an inaudible third (S3) and fourth (S4)
        heart sound.

3-19   The timing of a heart murmur helps in determining its cause. Systolic heart
murmurs are heard between the first (S1) and second (S2) heart sounds. They:

(a)   are always pathological
(b)   are usually due to mitral stenosis
(c)   may be due to mitral regurgitation if they are pansystolic
(d)   may be due to mitral valve prolapse
(e)   may be due to aortic stenosis if they are ejection systolic in character.

Photograph 3.3

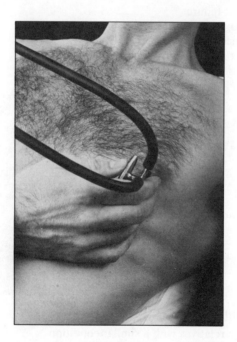

3-20   Listening with the bell of the stethoscope in the position shown in Photograph
3.3 is most helpful in the diagnosis of (choose the one best answer):

(a) mitral stenosis
(b) mitral regurgitation
(c) aortic stenosis
(d) aortic regurgitation
(e) pulmonary stenosis.

Photograph 3.4

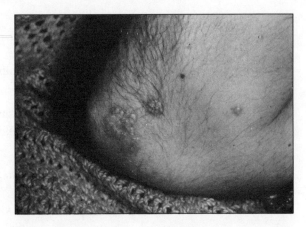

3-21 The patient in Photograph 3.4 is most likely to have (choose the one best answer):

(a) right heart failure
(b) severe aortic valve disease
(c) thyrotoxicosis
(d) raised serum cholesterol and triglyceride levels
(e) ankle oedema unilaterally.

Photograph 3.5

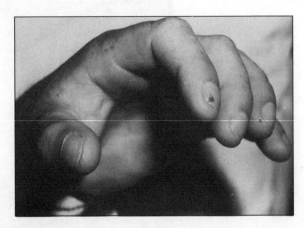

3-22 The patient in Photograph 3.5:

(a) may have relatives with a similar condition
(b) almost certainly has significant coronary artery disease
(c) has cardiomyopathy
(d) has hypertension
(e) has asthma.

3-23 A chest X-ray of a patient with severe mitral stenosis is most likely to show which one of the following (choose the one best answer):

  (a) left ventricular enlargement
  (b) left atrial enlargement
  (c) gross mitral valve calcification
  (d) a widening of the mediastinum
  (e) pulmonary plethora.

3-24 When one considers the X-ray of a patient with Marfan's syndrome, which of the following is most likely to be true (choose the one best answer)?

  (a) The left ventricle will be enlarged
  (b) The right ventricle will be enlarged
  (c) Aortic valve calcification will be present
  (d) The mediastinum may appear large if dilatation of the ascending aorta has occurred
  (e) There will be signs of left atrial dilatation.

3-25 The patient with normal atrioventricular conduction who presents with atrial fibrillation will *always* have which one of the following:

  (a) palpitations
  (b) an irregular pulse
  (c) tachycardia
  (d) cardiac failure
  (e) exertional dyspnoea.

3-26 The patient in Photograph 3.5 has presented with loss of weight and intermittent fever for over two months. Important questions to ask her about include:

  (a) a history of dental procedures in the preceding three months
  (b) the presence of any neurological symptoms of recent onset
  (c) a history of heart murmurs
  (d) a recent gastrointestinal procedure such as an oesophageal dilatation
  (e) a history of rheumatic fever in childhood.

3-27 When examining the patient in Photograph 3.5, other important signs to look for include:

  (a) haematuria
  (b) prosthetic valve sounds
  (c) absence of a peripheral pulse
  (d) ascites
  (e) a third heart sound (S3).

3-28 The most common cause of an abdominal bruit is (choose the one best answer):

  (a) renal failure
  (b) an innocent sound arising from the splenic artery
  (c) an abdominal aortic aneurysm
  (d) recent consumption of a large meal
  (e) a vascular liver tumour.

3-29   Continuous murmurs

   (a)   are always pathological
       because
   (b)   they are always due to an abnormal communication between two parts of
       the circulation.

3-30   Asking someone with suspected hypertrophic cardiomyopathy (HCM) to
squat may surprise the patient but will:

   (a)   increase the intensity of the systolic murmur
       because
   (b)   the outflow obstruction is decreased.

3-31   Making a correct diagnosis of cardiac failure is important because it is a serious
condition that may have a poor prognosis. Cardiac failure is present when the
cardiac output has fallen to the point where it no longer meets the needs of the
body. Patients with cardiac failure:

   (a)   are always hypotensive
   (b)   almost always have central cyanosis
   (c)   often have sinus tachycardia
   (d)   may have a palpable gallop rhythm
   (e)   may have mitral regurgitation secondary to mitral valve ring dilatation.

3-32   Right ventricular failure is difficult to diagnose unless more than one physical
sign is present. Patients with right ventricular failure:

   (a)   may complain of peripheral oedema
   (b)   have a raised jugular venous pressure (JVP) and large *v* waves, in many
       cases
   (c)   can reliably have tricuspid regurgitation excluded if no systolic murmur is
       present
   (d)   often have tender hepatomegaly due to hepatic infarction
   (e)   may develop ascites.

3-33   Myocardial infarction cannot usually be diagnosed with certainty from the
history or examination. If cases are not to be missed, it should be suspected
more often than it is finally diagnosed. A patient presenting with myocardial
infarction:

   (a)   may have no definite physical signs
   (b)   has an adverse prognosis if a third heart sound (S3) is present
   (c)   is at risk of developing atrial fibrillation, ventricular tachycardia or heart
       block
   (d)   who develops further chest pain has usually had further myocardial
       infarction
   (e)   is at risk of embolic stroke.

3-34 Infective endocarditis is a serious illness requiring aggressive treatment if the patient is to survive. There is often a long history and a rather gradual onset of symptoms. Patients with infective endocarditis:

    (a)   will always have a pre-existing valve lesion *esp of drug addict - on*
    (b)   may develop finger clubbing
    (c)   will usually have Osler's nodes present
    (d)   may have splinter haemorrhages
    (e)   may have a prosthetic heart valve.

3-35 A diagnosis of hypertension is important because the condition carries an adverse prognosis. Hypertensive patients:

    (a)   usually have a reversible cause for the hypertension that can be identified
    (b)   will often have a fourth heart sound (S4) if the diastolic blood pressure is greater than 110mmHg
    (c)   may develop papilloedema
    (d)   will usually have some symptoms due to the hypertension
    (e)   have an increased risk of developing cardiac failure if untreated.

3-36 Even though a specific underlying cause is not often found, there are a number of conditions associated with hypertension. Control of these may help control of the blood pressure. The following may be associated with or directly cause hypertension:

    (a)   obesity *1 stone ↓ in wt ↓ 6 mmHg.*
    (b)   moderate to heavy alcohol consumption
    (c)   smoking *NO*
    (d)   renal artery stenosis
    (e)   Cushing's syndrome.

3-37 As part of the examination of the patient who presents with dyspnoea, mitral stenosis should be excluded. Patients with mitral stenosis:

    (a)   are said to have severe disease if the valve area is less than 4cm^2 *—less than 1cm^2*
    (b)   have usually had rheumatic fever
    (c)   usually have a loud first heart sound (S1)
    (d)   usually have an early diastolic murmur
    (e)   are at increased risk of developing atrial fibrillation.

3-38 Patients with mitral valve prolapse are often asymptomatic and the condition may be detected during a routine examination. This condition:

    (a)   is common
    (b)   is always associated with a mid-systolic click
    (c)   is always associated with a late systolic murmur
    (d)   usually causes a considerably reduced life expectancy
    (e)   is now the most common cause of isolated mitral regurgitation.

3-39 Aortic stenosis may be suspected from the patient's history. The diagnosis should be made on physical examination. Patients with aortic stenosis:

(a)   may develop exertional syncope early in the disease
(b)   may have a systolic thrill palpable over the base of the heart
(c)   have always had rheumatic fever
(d)   rarely have associated aortic regurgitation
(e)   have an adverse prognosis if left ventricular failure has developed.

3-40   Aortic regurgitation may coexist with aortic stenosis or occur independently. There are a number of possible causes which can produce similar clinical signs. Aortic regurgitation:

(a)   often has a congenital aetiology
(b)   is associated with symptoms early in the course of the disease
(c)   is associated with a collapsing pulse
(d)   causes a characteristic decrescendo diastolic murmur
(e)   is usually well tolerated for long periods before cardiac failure supervenes.

3-41   The most common cause of mitral regurgitation in a patient who has no evidence of mitral stenosis is:

(a)   congenital
(b)   myocardial infarction with papillary muscle damage
(c)   mitral valve prolapse
(d)   rheumatic heart disease
(e)   secondary to aortic valve disease.

3-42   A patient who has had aortic valve replacement will always have:

(a)   a mechanical valve sound
(b)   a median sternotomy scar
(c)   coronary artery bypass grafting performed
(d)   signs of cardiac enlargement
(e)   the need to take an anticoagulant such as warfarin to protect from embolic events.

3-43   A patient with cardiomegaly will always have:

(a)   an increased cardiothoracic ratio on a chest X-ray film
(b)   exertional dyspnoea
(c)   a third heart sound (S3)
(d)   a fourth heart sound (S4)
(e)   a dilated cardiomyopathy.

3-44   Patients with dilated cardiomyopathy most commonly present with (choose the one best answer):

(a)   dyspnoea
(b)   chest pain
(c)   ankle oedema
(d)   fever
(e)   palpitations.

3-45 A patient with hypertension:

    (a)   will usually present with symptoms caused by the condition

    (b)   will not be able to reduce his or her blood pressure without drug treatment

    (c)   can have the diagnosis confirmed if a single blood pressure reading is as high as 160/95mmHg

    (d)   will usually not have an underlying identifiable cause or condition

    (e)   can always have the blood pressure controlled by a single drug.

Photograph 3.6

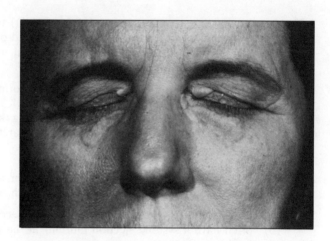

3-46 The patient in Photograph 3.6:

    (a)   will definitely have coronary artery disease

    (b)   will probably have a raised serum cholesterol level

    (c)   will probably have relatives with coronary artery disease

    (d)   may well have similar lesions over extensor tendons

    (e)   may have abnormal thyroid function.

3-47 In adults, pulmonary valve disease is less common than mitral and aortic valve disease. Patients with significant pulmonary stenosis:

    (a)   will have a soft systolic murmur

    (b)   often have a thrill palpable over the pulmonary area

    (c)   have a systolic murmur which is louder with inspiration

    (d)   usually have had rheumatic fever in the past

    (e)   may have a right ventricular fourth heart sound (S4).

3-48 Dilated cardiomyopathy is a very serious condition often associated with severe global dysfunction of the myocardium. Patients may present with dyspnoea and young patients are often misdiagnosed as having asthma or a viral illness. Signs of cardiac failure, however, are usually present. The following are considered causes of dilated cardiomyopathy:

- (a) viral myocarditis
- (b) aminoglycoside antibiotics
- (c) smoking
- (d) excessive alcohol consumption
- (e) dystrophia myotonica.

3-49 Acute aortic dissection:

- (a) may be associated with myocardial infarction
  because
- (b) dissection may extend into the origin of one of the coronary arteries.

3-50 A patient with a ventricular septal defect (VSD) may present with cardiac failure, but more often a murmur has been found on a routine examination. The characteristic signs of the condition should make the diagnosis fairly straightforward on physical examination. A VSD:

- (a) is the most common congenital cardiac abnormality
- (b) is usually associated with central cyanosis
- (c) is often associated with a systolic thrill along the mid-sternal edge
- (d) may be acquired following a myocardial infarction
- (e) may cause no symptoms throughout life.

3-51 Patients with an atrial septal defect (ASD) may present with a heart murmur first noticed on routine examination. Patients with an ASD:

- (a) usually have wide reversed splitting of the second heart sound (S2)
- (b) often have a systolic ejection murmur in the pulmonary area which is louder on inspiration
- (c) usually have a murmur of mitral regurgitation if the defect is a secundum defect
- (d) usually have fixed splitting of the second heart sound
- (e) may occasionally not present until middle age.

3-52 A patent ductus arteriosus:

- (a) is usually associated with a continuous murmur loudest below the left clavicle
  because
- (b) continuous shunting occurs from the descending aorta to the pulmonary artery.

3-53 Eisenmenger's syndrome:

- (a) is associated with central cyanosis
  because
- (b) left-to-right shunting of blood occurs between the pulmonary and systemic circulations.

3-54 Looking at the chest X-ray is considered an extension of the physical examination for patients with suspected cardiac or respiratory disease. With regard to the cardiac outline on the PA (posteroanterior) view:

 (a)   the right heart border is formed by the outer border of the right ventricle
 (b)   the aortic knuckle is usually present above the left hilum
 (c)   the heart is considered enlarged only when the cardiothoracic ratio exceeds 60%
 (d)   valve calcification is always present when a patient has significant valvular heart disease
 (e)   the hila outlines are formed mostly by the pulmonary arteries.

3-55   The diameter of the heart on the chest X-ray should be compared with the maximum width of the chest — the cardiothoracic ratio. Mild increases in this ratio may be present in patients with a reduced anteroposterior (AP) diameter of the chest, but possible pathological causes of an enlarged cardiac outline on chest X-ray include:

 (a)   left ventricular hypertrophy
 (b)   left ventricular dilatation
 (c)   right ventricular dilatation
 (d)   pericardial effusion
 (e)   dextrocardia.

Chapter 4

The Respiratory System and Breast Examination

Roses are red
Violets are blue
Without your lungs
Your blood would be too.

D D Ralph (*New England Journal of Medicine, 1981*)

4-1   An adult patient who presents with a dry cough which has been present for more than a few weeks:

   (a)   may have asthma
   (b)   is unlikely to have bronchiectasis
   (c)   may be taking an angiotensin-converting enzyme inhibitor
   (d)   may have cardiac failure
   (e)   may have cystic fibrosis.

4-2   Haemoptysis (or the coughing-up of blood) is an important presenting sign of respiratory disease. It frequently causes the patient great alarm so that medical advice is sought early. Causes of haemoptysis include:

   (a)   foreign body inhalation
   (b)   carcinoma of the lung
   (c)   pneumonia
   (d)   excessive alcohol intake
   (e)   pulmonary infarction.

4-3   Patients with dyspnoea may present first to a cardiologist or a respiratory physician. Even after history-taking and examination, the cause of the dyspnoea may not be clear. When a patient presents with dyspnoea:

   (a)   class IV symptoms mean the patient is breathless at rest
   (b)   asthma may be the cause even if there is no obvious wheeze
   (c)   cardiac failure should be considered a possible cause if the patient has paroxysmal nocturnal dyspnoea
   (d)   this is always due to either cardiac or respiratory disease
   (e)   it may be due to pulmonary embolism following a surgical operation.

4-4   Respiratory physicians take very detailed histories from their patients because of the large number of possible causes of respiratory disease. Patients may be puzzled at the relevance of some of the questions. However, when taking a respiratory patient's history:

   (a)   it may be useful to ask if the nextdoor neighbour has birds

(b) a patient's occupational dust exposure more than 10 years before is not relevant
(c) questions about eyedrops may be relevant
(d) the number of packet years of cigarette smoking should be asked about even if the patient has stopped smoking
(e) previous use of cytotoxic drugs may be relevant.

4-5 Patients with finger clubbing:

(a) may have tenderness over the wrists
because
(b) hypertrophic pulmonary osteoarthropathy is always present in patients with clubbing.

4-6 Staining of the fingers in cigarette smokers:

(a) is not a reliable sign of the number of cigarettes smoked
because
(b) nicotine is colourless.

4-7 Thoracoplasty:

(a) is a cause of severe chest deformity, but is not performed any more
because
(b) effective antimicrobial treatment for tuberculosis is available.

4-8 During the examination of a patient's chest, subcutaneous emphysema may be detected. Patients even occasionally notice this themselves. Subcutaneous emphysema:

(a) is a crackling sensation felt on palpating the skin of the chest or neck
(b) may be a normal finding
(c) may occasionally follow rupture of the oesophagus
(d) is most often due to a pneumothorax
(e) may occur following a thoracotomy.

4-9 A great deal of information can be gained from the assessment of a patient's chest wall movement. Time spent doing this carefully is well used and, of course, impresses examiners. When movement of the chest wall is being assessed:

(a) expansion of the upper lobes is best assessed from behind the patient
(b) lower lobe expansion is best assessed from in front of the patient
(c) reduced wall movement on one side is almost always due to lung collapse
(d) bilateral reduction in chest wall movement may occur with chronic air-flow limitation (chronic obstructive pulmonary disease)
(e) reduction of upper and lower lobe expansion may occur in pulmonary fibrosis.

4-10 Valuable information can often be obtained from percussion over various parts of the body. Accurate percussion requires practice and the percussion note should be felt as well as heard. During percussion over the chest and abdomen:

(a) a resonant note is usually heard over normal lungs
(b) a dull note is heard over fluid-filled areas such as a pleural effusion
(c) hyper-resonance is heard over bowel or pneumothorax
(d) a dull note is heard over an area of lung consolidation
(e) the upper border of the liver may be fairly accurately determined in most cases.

4-11 The stethoscope was invented by Laënnec so that doctors might avoid the embarrassment of listening to a patient's chest with their ears pressed up against the skin. Although fairly accurate auscultation can be performed the old way, it is usually recommended that the stethoscope be used. During auscultation of the chest:

(a) vesicular breath sounds are heard over normal lung
(b) vesicular breath sounds are louder and longer on inspiration than on expiration
(c) there is normally a gap between the inspiratory and expiratory sounds
(d) bronchial breath sounds are usually heard over areas of consolidation
(e) amphoric breath sounds may be heard over a cavity.

4-12 Breath sounds:

(a) should not be described in terms of air entry
because
(b) the entry of air into the lung cannot be directly gauged from the breath sounds.

4-13 It is simpler and more accurate to describe breath sounds as normal (vesicular), bronchial or reduced. Causes of reduced but not absent breath sounds include:

(a) consolidation
(b) pleural effusion
(c) emphysema
(d) listening over the main bronchi
(e) pneumothorax.

4-14 Wheezes (rhonchi) are continuous sounds. They:

(a) tend to be louder on inspiration
because
(b) pulmonary pressures are higher on inspiration.

4-15 There are many synonyms for the obstruction to movement of air caused by diseases of the airway. It is often reasonable to make a diagnosis of airflow limitation, although this does not indicate the aetiology. Patients with airflow limitation:

(a) may have this caused by asthma
(b) always have wheezes audible on auscultation of the chest
(c) usually have more severe obstruction if the wheezing is louder
(d) may have obstruction of a single bronchus causing a monophonic wheeze
(e) almost always complain of dyspnoea.

4-16   Continuous sounds heard on auscultation of the chest are often described as musical. There are also a number of non-musical sounds. Interrupted non-musical sounds that are heard on auscultation of the chest:

(a)   are usually called fine crackles (crepitations) if they are high pitched

(b)   are usually called low-pitched crackles (rales) if the sound is more coarse or lower pitched

(c)   pan-inspiratory crackles characteristically occur in chronic airflow limitation

(d)   fine inspiratory crackles caused by pulmonary fibrosis sound like Velcro

(e)   coarse crackles are a normal finding.

4-17   A friction rub is a sound which varies during the respiratory cycle. It tends to be effervescent (it is said to have usually disappeared by the time students can be found to come and listen). A patient with a friction rub:

(a)   may have pericarditis

(b)   may have pulmonary infarction

(c)   is very unlikely to have pneumonia

(d)   may have chest pain on deep inspiration

(e)   may have a palpable grating sensation over the same area.

4-18   Testing vocal resonance is a way of assessing underlying structures in the chest. Traditionally, the patient is asked to say '99' while the examiner listens over the chest. Some variety can be introduced by asking the patient to say "one one one". Getting a patient to say (or whisper) '99':

(a)   will accentuate high frequencies when the stethoscope is placed over consolidated lung

(b)   will make the speech more clearly audible over normal lung than consolidated lung

(c)   will enable you to detect vocal resonance in the area of a pleural effusion if this is present

(d)   may enable the detection of whispering pectoriloquy

(e)   will accentuate high frequencies when the stethoscope is placed over normal lung.

4-19   Lung disease may in some cases result in changes to the pulmonary vasculature, causing increases in systemic pressures in the pulmonary circulation that affect right ventricular function. Examining a respiratory patient for signs of pulmonary hypertension is important because:

(a)   this is commonly caused by pneumonia

(b)   may be a sign of pulmonary thromboembolism

(c)   can occur in pulmonary fibrosis

(d)   is common in patients with a lung abscess

(e)   may be a sign of pneumothorax.

4-20   A forced expiratory time of three seconds:

(a)   suggests chronic airflow imitation
      because
(b)   forced expiratory time is reduced in patients with chronic airways disease.

4-21   Peak flow meters are now readily available and should be used in the clinical assessment of the respiratory patient. Patients with chronic lung disease may have their own meters which they use at home. Measurements are of little use, however, unless the device is used correctly. The peak flow meter:

(a)   is used to measure the peak expiratory flow rate (PEFR)
(b)   in normal men will record approximately 600mL per minute PEFR
(c)   will reveal a high PEFR in patients with asthma
(d)   produces the most accurate reading when the patient gives a rapid expiratory puff
(e)   normal values depend on age, gender and height.

4-22   The spirometer is a more complicated device for assessing lung function but should be used in the bedside assessment of the dyspnoeic patient. The spirometer:

(a)   enables the measurement of the forced expiratory volume (FEV) and the forced expiratory volume in one second (FEV_1)
(b)   enables the measurement of the forced vital capacity (FVC)
(c)   readings should be taken three times and the average calculated
(d)   normally produces an FEV_1 to FVC ratio of 80% in young men
(e)   produces an FEV_1 to FVC ratio which increases with age.

4-23   A diagnosis of lobar pneumonia can often be made clinically. The following are important signs of consolidation:

(a)   a dull percussion note
(b)   vesicular breath sounds
(c)   an increased vocal resonance
(d)   increased expansion on the affected side
(e)   amphoric breath sounds.

4-24   The pleural space is a potential cavity between the visceral and thoracic layers of the pleura. Like the pericardial sac, it can become filled with various fluids. A collection of fluid in the pleural space:

(a)   may cause no symptoms
(b)   is called a haemothorax if it consists of blood
(c)   is called a chylothorax if it consists of pus
(d)   may have an area of bronchial breathing audible above it
(e)   always implies lung disease.

4-25   A pneumothorax:

(a)   may be associated with subcutaneous emphysema
      because
(b)   air has leaked into the subcutaneous tissues.

4-26   A patient who presents with the sudden onset of severe chest pain must be examined for signs of a pneumothorax. The diagnosis can often be suspected clinically. Spontaneous pneumothoraces are most common in young, tall, thin men. Signs of a pneumothorax include:

(a)   increased expansion on the affected side
(b)   reduced or absent breath sounds
(c)   a hyporesonant percussion note
(d)   hypotension if the pneumothorax is under tension
(e)   cyanosis in most cases.

4-27   A diagnosis of bronchiectasis can often be made on the basis of a careful history. Although this may not be altogether pleasant, examination of a patient's sputum cup, if available, is most important. Patients with bronchiectasis:

(a)   usually produce large amounts of purulent sputum
(b)   usually have a history of chronic cough and sputum production since childhood
(c)   almost always have finger clubbing
(d)   may have signs of airways obstruction
(e)   may have cystic fibrosis as the underlying abnormality.

4-28   The diagnosis of an acute asthma attack is usually straightforward. Appropriate treatment should be begun as quickly as possible. Severe asthma is a life-threatening disease. Signs of a severe asthma attack include:

(a)   a normally inflated chest
(b)   inability to speak because of dyspnoea
(c)   cyanosis
(d)   increased breath sounds
(e)   pulsus paradoxus of more than 20mmHg.

4-29   When examining patients with chronic lung disease, it is worth standing back and looking at the patient from a distance, since much information can be gained from general inspection. Patients with predominant emphysema:

(a)   usually look blue and bloated
(b)   may tend to breath through pursed lips
(c)   often need to use their accessory muscles of respiration
(d)   are usually smokers
(e)   usually have reduced expansion and underinflation of the chest.

4-30   Patients with pulmonary fibrosis:

(a)   have abnormal gas transfer
     because
(b)   there is ventilation-perfusion mismatching.

4-31   Pulmonary fibrosis is an important respiratory cause of dyspnoea. Diagnosis can in many cases be made on a physical examination and in some cases the aetiology may become apparent when the history is taken. Patients with pulmonary fibrosis:

    (a)   have almost always been cigarette smokers
    (b)   have often had exposure to mineral dusts
    (c)   do not develop finger clubbing
    (d)   typically have fine late inspiratory crackles at the bases of both lungs
    (e)   are more likely to have upper lobe fibrosis if the condition is associated with rheumatoid arthritis.

4-32 Tuberculosis is an important chronic respiratory disease which may present with a great variety of symptoms and signs. Patients with tuberculosis:

    (a)   are now very rarely seen in developed countries
    (b)   may have no abnormal chest signs
    (c)   typically complain of haemoptysis, night sweats and malaise
    (d)   may have erythema nodosum
    (e)   pose no threat of infection to other healthy people.

4-33 The structures in the mediastinum are rather important. They include the great vessels. Possible causes of mediastinal compression include:

    (a)   carcinoma of the lung
    (b)   emphysema
    (c)   dermoid cyst
    (d)   a large goitre
    (e)   penetrating chest injury without a pneumothorax.

4-34 The diagnosis of superior vena caval (SVC) obstruction may be suspected from a general inspection of the patient, but certain specific clinical signs should be sought. Patients with superior vena caval obstruction:

    (a)   may have exophthalmos
    (b)   should be examined for supraclavicular lymphadenopathy
    (c)   may have stridor from recurrent laryngeal nerve involvement
    (d)   should be examined for a Horner's syndrome
    (e)   typically have a low jugular venous pressure.

4-35 Patients with carcinoma of the lung:

    (a)   may have lethargy and confusion secondary to hyponatraemia
         because
    (b)   antidiuretic hormone is usually released by squamous cell carcinomas.

4-36 Sarcoidosis is one of the great disease imitators. Most parts of the body can be affected. Patients with sarcoidosis:

    (a)   have non-caseating granulomas which contain atypical mycobacteria
    (b)   have non-caseating granulomas which are found only in the lungs
    (c)   may develop pulmonary fibrosis
    (d)   may develop violaceous patches on the nose or fingers called lupus pernio
    (e)   usually have splenomegaly.

4-37   Pulmonary embolism is an important and common condition which is often underdiagnosed. Certain physical signs may provide helpful clues to the diagnosis. Pulmonary embolism:

(a)   is a cause of sudden death
(b)   may cause no symptoms
(c)   is more common in immobilised patients
(d)   may present with dyspnoea and haemoptysis
(e)   may cause chronic right ventricular failure.

4-38   An examination of the breast should be a routine part of the physical examination in women. Carcinoma of the breast is a common malignancy in women and also occasionally occurs in men. In examination of the breasts:

(a)   nipple retraction on one side is almost always an indication of underlying malignancy
(b)   oedema of the skin secondary to carcinoma may cause a *peau d'orange* appearance
(c)   Paget's disease of the nipple is commonly due to infection
(d)   examination of the draining supraclavicular and axillary lymph nodes is part of the normal examination
(e)   mammary duct ectasia may be suspected when green fluid can be expressed from the nipple.

Photograph 4.1

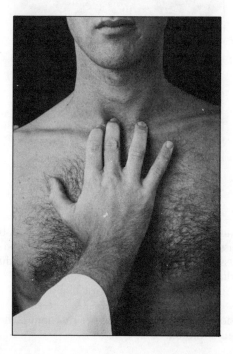

4-39   Palpation for the position of the trachea is an important part of the respiratory examination. One should begin as shown in Photograph 4.1:

(a)   it is necessary to push the examining finger back forcefully before one can decide if the trachea is in the normal position
(b)   the trachea may normally lie somewhat to the right or left of the midline above the suprasternal notch
(c)   changes in the position of the trachea are associated with changes in the upper lobes of the lung
(d)   in the Photograph 4.1, the examiner's fingers are placed correctly for the detection of a tracheal tug
(e)   getting a patient to drink a glass of water while feeling the trachea may assist in its assessment.

Photograph 4.2

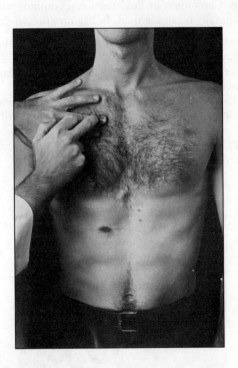

4-40   In Photograph 4.2:

(a)   the examiner is percussing over the right middle lobe
(b)   the percussion note in this area should normally be resonant
(c)   the percussion note at this level on the left side is dull because of under-lying cardiac structures
(d)   a dull percussion note here is most likely due to a right-sided pleural effusion
(e)   a percussion note here may be hyper-resonant if the patient has a right-sided pneumothorax.

4-41 In Photograph 4.3:

  (a) the examiner is attempting to assess lower lobe expansion
  (b) the examiner has his thumbs correctly placed to compare right and left sided movement
  (c) reduced movement of one side suggests pathology on the other side
  (d) detection of reduced expansion on both sides is consistent with pulmonary fibrosis
  (e) increased expansion on both sides suggests chronic airflow limitation.

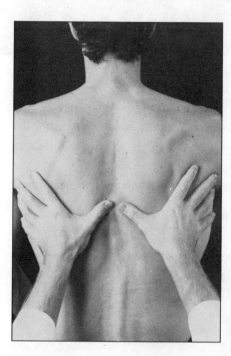

Photograph 4.3

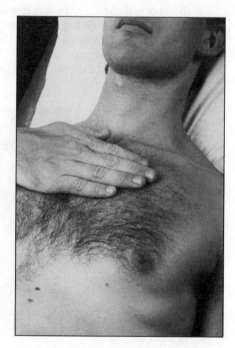

Photograph 4.4

4-42 The examiner in Photograph 4.4:

  (a) is feeling for a displaced apex beat
  (b) may be able to detect evidence of pulmonary hypertension
  (c) may feel a diastolic thrill if the patient has a ventricular septal defect
  (d) may feel a systolic thrill if the patient has pulmonary stenosis
  (e) is unlikely to be able to feel subcutaneous emphysema in this position.

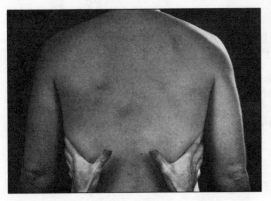

Photograph 4.5

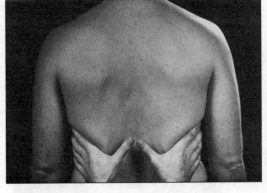

Photograph 4.6

4-43   In Photographs 4.5 and 4.6:

   (a)   the examiner's thumbs have lost contact with the chest wall, reducing the value of the examination
   (b)   normal chest expansion appears to be present
   (c)   the examiner's fingers are clubbed
   (d)   reduced movement of the thumbs is likely if the patient has chronic airflow limitation
   (e)   reduction in expansion may occur on the affected side if the patient has consolidation.

Photograph 4.7

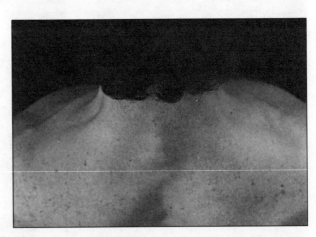

4-44   In Photograph 4.7:

   (a)   this patient is well positioned for assessment of upper lobe expansion
   (b)   reduced movement of both clavicles is consistent with upper lobe fibrosis
   (c)   reduced movement of the right clavicle may occur with a right-sided pleural effusion
   (d)   supraclavicular lymphadenopathy is usually well seen in this position
   (e)   movement of the clavicles is normally slightly asymmetrical because of the position of the heart on the left side.

4-45 Sarcoidosis is a systemic disease. Involvement is most common in (choose the one best answer):

    (a)   liver and spleen
    (b)   the carotids
    (c)   the heart leading to heart block
    (d)   the lungs
    (e)   the eyes.

4-46 The most common cause of chronic bronchitis is (choose the one best answer):

    (a)   air pollution
    (b)   exposure to factory dusts
    (c)   cystic fibrosis
    (d)   smoking
    (e)   recurrent aspiration pneumonia.

4-47 A cough is a very common presenting symptom. The presence of a dry repetitive cough:

    (a)   may be a sign of asthma
    (b)   is always pathological
    (c)   is a common symptom of bronchiectasis
    (d)   is almost never a sign of cardiac failure
    (e)   may be related to the use of certain antibiotics.

4-48 Patients with metabolic acidosis (for example, in diabetes mellitus or chronic renal failure) may present with Kussmaul's breathing. This pattern of breathing is most commonly (choose the one best answer):

    (a)   irregular in timing and depth
    (b)   deep and rapid
    (c)   characterised by a post-inspiratory pause
    (d)   characterised by periods of apnoea alternating with hyperpnoea
    (e)   similar to the disturbed breathing of patients with sleep apnoea.

4-49 A patient who has had radiotherapy to the chest for a carcinoma of the lung or lymphoma will have chest wall changes related to this treatment. The most common finding is (choose the one best answer):

    (a)   decreased pigmentation in the irradiated area
    (b)   the presence of permanent subcutaneous emphysema
    (c)   the presence of erythema and thickening with a sharp demarcation
    (d)   the presence of large tattooed lines marking out the entire extent of the area irradiated
    (e)   wasting of the chest wall muscles on that side.

4-50 The examination of the chest X-ray is an extension of the physical examination. The most common cause for a reverse position of the apex of the heart is (choose the one best answer):

    (a)   cardiac enlargement
    (b)   dextrocardia
    (c)   incorrect left and right markings on the X-ray film
    (d)   a left-sided pneumothorax
    (e)   severe mitral valve disease.

4-51 The shadows of a number of structures visible on X-ray make up the left border of the heart. Which one of the following is *not* part of this silhouette (choose the one best answer):

    (a)   the left ventricular apex
    (b)   the left atrial appendage
    (c)   the left main bronchus
    (d)   the left main pulmonary artery
    (e)   the aortic knuckle.

Chapter 5

The Gastrointestinal System

I don't have ulcers; I give them.

Harry Cohn (1891–1958)

5-1 A 30-year-old man presents to see you with a two-month history of burning epigastric pain that wakes him from sleep at night and is relieved by eating. He describes no heartburn, acid regurgitation, vomiting, weight loss, bowel disturbance or other complaints. Which of the following conditions is most likely to explain his symptoms (choose the one best answer):

(a) irritable bowel syndrome
(b) peptic ulcer disease
(c) oesophageal adenocarcinoma
(d) carcinoma of the colon
(e) gallstones.

5-2 An increased appetite associated with substantial weight loss can occur in which of the following disease states?

(a) thyrotoxicosis
(b) lung cancer
(c) depression
(d) pancreatic cancer
(e) anorexia nervosa.

5-3 Odynophagia (painful swallowing) often occurs in which of the following conditions:

(a) oesophageal obstruction with a cancer
(b) oesophageal ulceration
(c) following ingestion of caustic substances
(d) immunosuppressed patients with herpes simplex oesophagitis
(e) *Candida* oesophagitis.

5-4 In the patient with steatorrhoea which of the following is/are correct?

(a) The stools are typically very pale, malodorous and difficult to flush away
(b) Malabsorption of the fat-soluble vitamins (A, D, E and K) occurs
(c) Examination of the skin is unhelpful
(d) Previous upper abdominal surgery may be a cause
(e) The mouth should be inspected.

5-5 A 50-year-old woman taking non-steroidal anti-inflammatory drugs for rheumatoid arthritis presents with a history of dark black stools over the past week and feelings of lethargy. On physical examination she has pallor of the palmar creases and pale conjunctivae. The following most likely explains her complaints (select the one best answer):

  (a) bismuth ingestion
  (b) haemorrhoids
  (c) anal fissure
  (d) peptic ulcer
  (e) aphthous ulceration of the mouth.

5-6 Which of the following skin and gut conditions are associated?

  (a) Pigmented macules on lips — benign bowel polyps
  (b) Vesicles on hands — liver disease
  (c) Flushing — carcinoid tumour
  (d) Itchy vesicles on knees and elbows — malabsorption
  (e) Brown papillomas in the axillae — gastro-oesophageal reflux.

5-7 White nails are found in:

  (a) chronic liver disease
  (b) fever
  (c) bowel cancer
  (d) porphyria cutanea tarda
  (e) thyrotoxicosis.

5-8 Signs of chronic liver disease include:

  (a) palmar erythema
  (b) asterixis
  (c) Dupuytren's contractures
  (d) scleral icterus
  (e) spider naevi.

5-9 Moderate to massive hepatomegaly can be caused by:

  (a) alcoholic cirrhosis in the absence of fatty infiltration
  (b) heart failure
  (c) gallstones in the gallbladder
  (d) non-metastatic colonic cancer
  (e) caput Medusae.

5-10 Hepatosplenomegaly may typically occur with:

  (a) portal hypertension and chronic liver disease
  (b) metastatic involvement of the liver by colonic cancer
  (c) lymphoma
  (d) infectious mononucleosis
  (e) leukaemia.

5-11 A thin inactive 75-year-old man presents to hospital for a right inguinal hernia repair. During your routine physical examination, you feel a mass in the left iliac fossa that is non-tender and non-pulsatile but indents on being pressed firmly. Rectal examination is normal except for firm stool in the vault. The most likely diagnosis is (select the one best answer):

(a) left colonic cancer
(b) a colonic polyp
(c) stool
(d) an aortic aneurysm
(e) a diverticular abscess.

5-12 During the abdominal examination it may be necessary to look for shifting dullness. The term means:

(a) the examiner is too dull to shift the patient
(b) movement of the liver can be assessed during respiration
(c) shifting patients is dull
(d) when the patient rolls towards the examiner, dullness in the flank becomes resonant
(e) a fluid thrill is present over the liver.

5-13 Causes of abdominal distension include:

(a) ascites
(b) irritable bowel syndrome
(c) severe constipation
(d) pregnancy
(e) pelvic tumour.

5-14 The inability to hear bowel sounds on auscultation of the abdomen suggests:

(a) the patient is not fasting
(b) an insufficiently expensive stethoscope has been used
(c) a friction rub is present
(d) intestinal hurry
(e) paralytic ileus.

5-15 Rectal examination:

(a) is *not* a routine part of the physical examination
(b) cannot be used to examine the prostate gland
(c) detects the cervix on the posterior wall of the rectum
(d) may detect occult rectal cancer if a mass is felt in the bowel wall
(e) is of no value in the patient with diarrhoea.

5-16   Which of the following is correct?

    (a)   In patients with haemolysis one would expect to find a raised urobilinogen

    (b)   In cases of obstructive jaundice with complete bile duct obstruction one would expect to find in the urine a raised conjugated bilirubin but absent urobilinogen

    (c)   Patients with viral hepatitis do not become jaundiced

    (d)   Patients with hepatocellular jaundice never have raised urobilinogen levels

    (e)   Stercobilin can be tested for in the urine.

5-17   Dysphagia:

    (a)   means painful swallowing

    (b)   may be associated with odynophagia

    (c)   is *not* a complication of gastro-oesophageal reflux

    (d)   *cannot* result from a large goitre

    (e)   is usually due to stress.

5-18   Hepatic encephalopathy:

    (a)   is a sign of liver failure

    (b)   is characterised by a fine regular tremor

    (c)   occurs with barbiturate overdose

    (d)   causes jaundice

    (e)   causes Dupuytren's contractures.

5-19   Steatorrhoea can be due to all of the following except (choose the one best answer):

    (a)   coeliac disease

    (b)   gastrectomy

    (c)   chronic pancreatitis

    (d)   ulcerative proctitis

    (e)   Crohn's disease.

5-20   Systemic signs of inflammatory bowel disease include:

    (a)   erythema nodosum

    (b)   clubbing

    (c)   iritis

    (d)   non-deforming arthritis

    (e)   cardiac failure.

5-21   A 45-year-old man presents with haematemesis and melaena. On examination, the lesions pictured in Photograph 5.1 (a and b) are found on his lips and tongue. Which of the following is/are correct?

    (a)   His relatives may also have these lesions

    (b)   He is likely to have signs of chronic liver disease

    (c)   This is called the Peutz-Jeghers syndrome

    (d)   He may be bleeding from telangiectasia in the small intestine

    (e)   His nail beds may be affected.

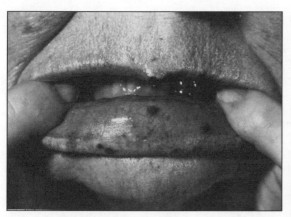

Photograph 5.1a

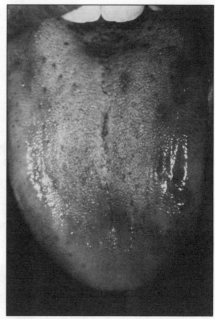

Photograph 5.1b

5-22 The possible causes of the patient's problem in Photograph 5.2 may include:

    (a)   portal hypertension
    (b)   hepatic vein thrombosis
    (c)   malignancy
    (d)   cholecystitis
    (e)   diverticulitis.

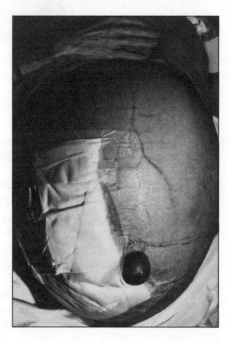

Photograph 5.2

5-23   Causes of a mass in the right groin of a male patient could include:

    (a)   femoral hernia
    (b)   direct inguinal hernia
    (c)   lymph node
    (d)   undescended testis
    (e)   lipoma.

5-24   A 50-year-old man on examination has clubbing, leuconychia, palmar ery-thema, multiple spider naevi, and shifting dullness on percussion of the abdo-men. The liver is impalpable. The cause of this man's physical signs is most likely to be (choose the one best answer):

    (a)   liver cirrhosis
    (b)   nephrotic syndrome
    (c)   metastatic liver disease
    (d)   hypothyroidism (myxoedema)
    (e)   pancreatitis.

Photograph 5.3

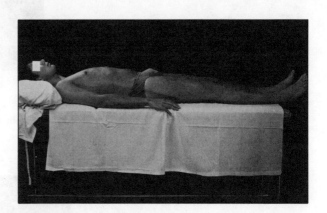

5-25   Photograph 5.3 shows the best position for examination:

    (a)   of hepatic encephalopathy
    (b)   of the abdomen
    (c)   with the sigmoidoscope
    (d)   of an indirect inguinal hernia
    (e)   of an initially impalpable spleen.

5-26   Examination of the gastrointestinal contents can provide clues about underly-ing disease. Which of the following statements are correct?

    (a)   Melaena stools indicate that bleeding may have occurred from anywhere in the colon
    (b)   Very pale, offensive, bulky stools suggest fat malabsorption
    (c)   Coffee ground vomitus is usually a result of recent coffee ingestion and is not of concern
    (d)   Haematochezia means that bright red blood has been passed per rectum and is always the result of anorectal pathology
    (e)   Bismuth can cause black stools.

5-27   Causes of a palpable liver include:

   (a)   emphysema
   (b)   Riedel's lobe
   (c)   right subphrenic abscess
   (d)   chronic constrictive pericarditis
   (e)   hydatid disease.

5-28   Testing the stools for blood using the guaiac test can be performed as part of the physical examination. This test:

   (a)   does not produce false-positive results
   (b)   is diagnostic of colorectal carcinoma if positive
   (c)   is not affected by the diet
   (d)   is recommended for population-based screening for colonic cancer in asymptomatic adults under the age of 40 years
   (e)   is useful in the physical examination of a patient with suspected anaemia.

5-29   On examining the mouth, you observe creamy white patches that can be scraped off only with difficulty. Which of the following is/are likely to be true in this case?

   (a)   HIV infection may be present
   (b)   The urine should be tested for sugar
   (c)   The fingernails and toenails should be examined
   (d)   The patient may have dysphagia
   (e)   The patient may have signs of alcoholism.

5-30   On abdominal palpation, you feel a mass in the left hypochondrium. There is a space between the mass and the left costal margin. The mass moves inferiorly on inspiration. Which of the following is correct?

   (a)   You should try to ballot the mass
   (b)   You should percuss over the mass to determine if it is resonant
   (c)   If a friction rub is audible over the mass, this suggests it is a kidney
   (d)   The mass is likely to be due to a gastric carcinoma
   (e)   The mass is likely to be a pancreatic pseudocyst.

5-31   When a skilled clinician or senior medical student examines a normal abdomen:

   (a)   a small amount of ascites can usually be detected
   (b)   the edge of the liver should not be palpable at all below the right costal margin
   (c)   it should not be possible to feel the spleen
   (d)   bowel sounds should only be audible for four hours after the patient has eaten
   (e)   a succussion splash should not be audible no matter how hard the examiner shakes the patient.

5-32   When a patient with duodenal ulceration is examined:

    (a)   one would not expect ever to find even mild epigastric tenderness
    (b)   the presence of clubbing is an unusual but important sign of the disease
    (c)   there are often no physical signs
    (d)   the rectal examination will usually reveal tenderness
    (e)   the characteristic skin rash of *Helicobacter pylori* infection will often be seen.

5-33   The following diagnoses may be suspected when a patient's breath is sampled:

    (a)   diabetic ketoacidosis
    (b)   vitamin B_{12} deficiency
    (c)   uraemia
    (d)   cigarette smoking
    (e)   oesophageal reflux.

5-34   In the assessment of patients with gastrointestinal bleeding:

    (a)   the presence of hypotension suggests that at least half the blood volume has been lost
    (b)   if bright red blood is passed per rectum, bleeding must have occurred from the large bowel
    (c)   the presence of melaena means enough blood has been lost to warrant transfusion
    (d)   a history of the ingestion of non-steroidal anti-inflammatory drugs may be relevant
    (e)   patients should be asked about recent symptoms of angina.

5-35   Inspection of the mouths of patients with malabsorption may be very rewarding. The following may be observed:

    (a)   purpura
    (b)   leucoplakia
    (c)   aphthous ulcers
    (d)   lingua nigra (black tongue)
    (e)   macroglossia.

5-36   Enlargement of the male breasts (gynaecomastia) has numerous causes. These include:

    (a)   use of the drug cimetidine
    (b)   chronic hepatitis
    (c)   carcinoma of the colon
    (d)   inflammatory bowel disease
    (e)   rheumatoid arthritis.

5-37   When the gallbladder is enlarged it may be palpable in the right hypochondrium. The following are possible causes of enlargement:

(a) carcinoma of the head of the pancreas
(b) carcinoma of the gallbladder
(c) severe hepatic cirrhosis
(d) chronic hepatitis
(e) chronic cholelithiasis.

5-38 Patients with ulcerative colitis may develop any of a number of skin changes. These include:

(a) erythema nodosum
(b) pyoderma gangrenosum
(c) areas of hyperpigmentation
(d) areas of hypopigmentation
(e) ichthyosis.

5-39 Toxic dilatation of the colon is an uncommon complication of ulcerative colitis. Signs of this condition include:

(a) abdominal distension
(b) jaundice
(c) abdominal guarding and rigidity
(d) fever and tachycardia
(e) clubbing.

5-40 The prostate gland:

(a) is not normally palpable when a rectal examination is performed on men below the age of 40 years
  because
(b) the gland only becomes palpable as it enlarges in old age.

Chapter 6

The Genitourinary System

Sex is one of the nine reasons for reincarnation.
The other eight are unimportant.

Henry Miller (1891–1980)

6-1 A red discoloration of the urine:

  (a) does not always not always imply haematuria
       because
  (b) this discoloration has other causes including consumption of large
       amounts of beetroot.

6-2 In the assessment of suspected urinary obstruction, the history must be taken
with some care. Patients with urinary obstruction:

  (a) are commonly elderly men with prostatic enlargement
  (b) may have difficulty starting micturition
  (c) may develop urinary incontinence
  (d) do not usually experience pain if the obstruction is due to ureteric calculi
  (e) frequently have nocturia.

6-3 A patient who presents feeling generally unwell with tiredness and lethargy
may only have a minor temporary illness. However, the onset of renal failure
can present this way. Patients with uraemia (chronic renal failure):

  (a) always have oliguria (less than 400mL of urine a day)
  (b) often have nocturia
  (c) may present with vomiting
  (d) can have skin problems including pruritus, bruising and oedema
  (e) are usually hypotensive.

6-4 Patients with a myocardial infarction and cardiogenic shock:

  (a) are at risk of acute renal failure
       because
  (b) release of large amounts of creatine kinase from the damaged
       myocardium can injure the kidneys.

6-5 Patients with chronic renal failure:

  (a) often have a sallow complexion
       because
  (b) there is iron deposition in the skin.

6-6 After making a general inspection of a patient with possible chronic renal failure, it is well worth spending some time on the fingernails. Fingernail changes may include:

(a) leuconychia related to hypoalbuminaemia
(b) clubbing
(c) half-and-half nails
(d) Mee's lines
(e) onycholysis.

6-7 Examination of the arms, in patients with chronic renal failure, may commonly reveal:

(a) bruising
(b) uraemic frost
(c) scratch marks
(d) skin pigmentation due to urochrome deposition
(e) areas of depigmentation.

6-8 Abdominal examination forms an important part of the assessment of the renal patient. When examining the abdomen:

(a) it is normal to be able to feel the lower poles of both kidneys in some thin patients
(b) transplanted kidneys are rarely palpable
(c) nephrectomy scars when present are in a posterior position
(d) an enlarged spleen may be confused with a palpable left kidney
(e) bilateral enlargement of the kidneys is often due to polycystic kidneys or hydronephrosis.

Photograph 6.1

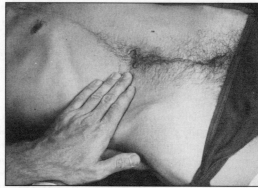

6-9 In Photograph 6.1 the right kidney is being ballotted:

(a) when this is done correctly, the examiner's hands are squeezed together until the kidney becomes palpable
(b) the fingers of the right hand are flexed briskly so that the right kidney floats upwards to be felt by the eagerly awaiting left hand
(c) a normal right kidney is never palpable
(d) an attempt should be made to ballot the liver in this position, as a matter of routine
(e) a kidney transplanted on the right side is also examined in this way.

Photograph 6.2

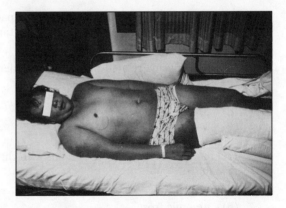

6-10   The patient in Photograph 6.2 has suffered severe injuries to his right leg and back. Likely causes of acute renal failure in this patient would include:

    (a)   hypovolaemia
    (b)   myoglobinaemia
    (c)   severe hypertension
    (d)   uncomplicated pelvic fracture
    (e)   small pulmonary embolus.

6-11   Patients with renal failure may have a visibly distended abdomen on examination because:

    (a)   this occurs in patients having peritoneal dialysis but only for a few hours since the fluid is rapidly absorbed
    (b)   large polycystic kidneys may occasionally cause abdominal distension
    (c)   most patients with renal failure have ascites
    (d)   bilateral renal transplants may make the abdomen appear distended
    (e)   of the presence of ascites which is diagnostic of hepatic failure.

6-12   Examination of the back is important in a patient with renal failure. Which of the following statements are correct?

    (a)   The patient may be surprised at the use of the clenched fist to strike the renal angle; this may elicit renal tenderness in patients with renal infection
    (b)   Patients with glomerulonephritis never develop oedema
    (c)   Striking the vertebral column with the base of the fist may elicit tenderness in patients with osteomalacia
    (d)   Nephrectomy scars may be visible posteriorly but not anteriorly
    (e)   Both kidneys are often palpable posteriorly.

6-13   In a patient with renal failure, examination of the rectum is important because:

    (a)   carcinoma of the rectum is a common cause of renal failure because of secondaries to the kidneys
    (b)   the enlarged bladder may be palpable in patients with hydronephrosis
    (c)   hard faeces in the rectum suggesting constipation is a useful sign of renal impairment

(d)   benign prostatic hyperplasia or prostatic carcinoma may be a cause of urinary obstruction

(e)   the ureters are sometimes palpable on rectal examination.

6-14   On examination of the legs:

(a)   most patients with renal failure will be found to have peripheral oedema

(b)   the presence of gouty tophi is common in patients with hyperuricaemia due to renal failure

(c)   the presence of tophi may suggest a cause for the patient's renal failure

(d)   peripheral neuropathy may occur

(e)   the presence of scratch marks suggests acute but not chronic renal failure.

6-15   A patient is found on examination to have bilaterally enlarged and irregular kidneys. The following symptoms or signs may also be present:

(a)   severe headache

(b)   hepatic or splenic cysts

(c)   bilateral carotid bruits

(d)   hypertension

(e)   proximal muscle weakness.

6-16   Examination and testing of the urine is an extension of the physical examination of the genitourinary system. Normal urine may smell:

(a)   of recently ingested asparagus

(b)   like fish

(c)   ammoniacal

(d)   of recently ingested antibiotics

(e)   like port wine.

6-17   The colour of urine is not examined with the intensity that it used to be, but certain information can be gained by this inspection:

(a)   colourless urine suggests excessive drinking or diabetes insipidus

(b)   red discoloration is always due to haematuria

(c)   severe haemoglobinuria make cause black discoloration of the urine as in blackwater fever

(d)   urine colour is not affected by diet

(e)   bacterial infection may cause clouding of the urine.

6-18   Chemical testing of the urine can be very useful:

(a)   when testing with a dipstick, a + of proteinuria is always abnormal

(b)   the presence of immunoglobulin light chains (Bence Jones proteinuria) can be excluded by chemical dipstick testing

(c)   glycosuria (the presence of sugar in the urine) is often a normal finding

(d)   the presence of ketones in the urine of diabetic patients suggests diabetic ketoacidosis

(e)   strip colour tests are equally sensitive to acetone and acetoacetic acid.

6-19   If a patient presents with proteinuria the following suggests the nephrotic syndrome:

(a)   hyperalbuminaemia
(b)   hypolipidaemia
(c)   proteinuria less than 3.5g per 24 hours
(d)   large palpable kidneys
(e)   peripheral oedema.

6-20   The examination of the urinary sediment:

(a)   should be on a first morning urine sample if possible
because
(b)   the urine is likely to be more concentrated.

6-21   Part of the examination of a patient with a scrotal mass is testing for translucency using a torch. A mass which is part of the testis, but not translucent, is most likely to be (choose the one best answer):

(a)   hard to see
(b)   a syphilitic gumma
(c)   a cyst of the epididymis
(d)   a tumour
(e)   an inguinoscrotal hernia.

6-22   The most common cause of a bloody vaginal discharge is (choose the one best answer):

(a)   carcinoma of the cervix
(b)   cervical polyp
(c)   vaginitis
(d)   a miscarriage
(e)   menstruation.

6-23   In a normal pelvic examination:

(a)   the cervix can be felt pointing towards the anterior vaginal wall
(b)   the ovaries are usually palpable
(c)   the uterus can normally be felt by bimanual palpation with one hand in the vagina and the other above the pubic symphysis
(d)   the most common cause of smooth enlargement of the uterus is pregnancy
(e)   the normal uterus is tender to palpation.

Chapter 7

The Haematological System

A disease known is half cured.

Proverb

7-1 A patient who presents with anaemia, particularly if iron deficiency is suspected, should be asked about which of the following as possible causes of blood loss:

    (a)   symptoms of peptic ulceration
    (b)   rectal bleeding
    (c)   melaena
    (d)   early menopause
    (e)   repeated blood donations.

7-2 Which one of the following is *unlikely* to be a symptom of anaemia (choose the one best answer):

    (a)   weakness
    (b)   lethargy
    (c)   easy bruising
    (d)   exertional dyspnoea
    (e)   fatigue.

7-3 It may be possible to get an idea of the cause of anaemia if a careful past history is taken from the patient. Relevant questions include:

    (a)   a history of aspirin use
    (b)   a history of malignancy
    (c)   a history of rheumatoid arthritis
    (d)   previous gastric surgery
    (e)   recent change in bowel patterns.

7-4 A patient receiving vitamin B_{12} may have pernicious anaemia. Pernicious anaemia:

    (a)   may occur in very strict vegetarians
    (b)   causes a microcytosis on blood film
    (c)   will probably have been treated with vitamin B_{12} tablets
    (d)   is a less common cause of anaemia than iron deficiency
    (e)   is usually treated by dietary supplementation with huge amounts of liver.

7-5 During the examination of the patient with a suspected haematological disease the general appearance is important. The following should be looked for during this examination:

(a)   the patient's racial origin
(b)   the presence of jaundice
(c)   the presence of scratch marks
(d)   the presence of obesity
(e)   the presence of polyarthritis.

7-6   Examination of the hands is useful in the assessment of a patient with suspected haematological disease or anaemia because:

(a)   the presence of koilonychia is only caused by iron deficiency anaemia
(b)   nail bed pallor is always due to significant anaemia
(c)   pallor of the palmar creases means the haemoglobin is always less than 70g per litre
(d)   in an anaemic patient with rheumatoid arthritis, it is useful to examine the spleen
(e)   the presence of gouty tophi in the hands is always an incidental finding.

7-7   Petechiae are pinhead-sized haemorrhages visible on the skin. Causes of petechiae include:

(a)   immunological damage to platelets in immune thrombocytopenic purpura (ITP)
(b)   platelet dysfunction caused by chronic renal failure
(c)   platelet dysfunction caused by paracetamol
(d)   sequestration of platelets in patients with hypersplenism
(e)   meningococcal septicaemia.

7-8   Ecchymoses are larger areas of subcutaneous bleeding. In the elderly patient the most common cause is (choose the one best answer):

(a)   Christmas disease (haemophilia B)
(b)   recent aspirin ingestion
(c)   loss of skin elasticity
(d)   haemophilia A
(e)   chronic liver disease.

7-9   There are three relatively common congenital bleeding disorders:

(a)   haemophilia B is called Christmas disease because it was discovered by a physician called Christmas
(b)   Christmas disease is due to factor IX deficiency
(c)   Von Willebrand's disease is the most severe of the congenital clotting disorders
(d)   haemophilia A is due to factor VIII deficiency
(e)   these congenital disorders more often present with haemorrhage than with bruising.

7-10   Examination of the lymph nodes is an important part of the haematological assessment:

(a) the normal position of the epitrochlear nodes is just anterior to the lateral epicondyle
(b) tender enlargement of an epitrochlear node is most commonly due to infection in the hand or arm
(c) the para-aortic lymph nodes are not usually palpable
(d) lymph nodes larger than 1cm in diameter are usually pathological
(e) lymph nodes larger than 1cm in diameter are almost always due to malignant disease.

7-11 The character of a palpable lymph node may suggest its aetiology:

(a) very hard nodes are often present in the inguinal region because of repeated infections in the feet and legs
(b) nodes with a rubbery consistency occur in lymphoma
(c) fixation of nodes to underlying structures suggests malignancy
(d) overlying inflammation of the skin suggests advanced malignancy
(e) the presence of firm palpable lymph nodes in the axilla in a woman with carcinoma of the breast suggests that the malignancy has spread to at least the regional nodes.

7-12 When examining a patient with suspected anaemia:

(a) it is important to look at the conjunctivae for pallor
because
(b) this is a more reliable sign of anaemia than pallor elsewhere.

7-13 Examination of the gums is important in suspected haematological disease because:

(a) gum hypertrophy is common in patients with anaemia
(b) acute monocytic leukaemia is associated with gum atrophy
(c) swollen and bleeding gums are characteristic of scurvy
(d) gum ulceration may be due to haematological disease but is more often due to badly fitting false teeth
(e) infection of the gums may occur in patients with a compromised immune system.

7-14 Examination for bony tenderness may surprise the patient, but it is important in a number of conditions:

(a) examination may be carried out by tapping over the spine with the fist
(b) striking the spine too hard is likely to elicit tenderness in even normal and stoical people
(c) the presence of tenderness is diagnostic of enlargement of the marrow due to infiltration by myeloma
(d) pressing the sternum with the heel of the hand is a useful way of eliciting the sign
(e) the presence of secondary malignant deposits in bone may cause areas of extreme tenderness.

7-15   The following are causes of generalised lymphadenopathy:

    (a)   lymphoma
    (b)   infectious mononucleosis
    (c)   sarcoidosis
    (d)   the drug digoxin
    (e)   systemic lupus erythematosus.

7-16   The presence of leg ulcers is an important sign of haematological disease. There are a number of possible causes of leg ulcers. The problem may relate to increased blood viscosity and tissue infarction in some cases. Associations with leg ulcers include:

    (a)   thalassaemia
    (b)   polycythaemia
    (c)   sickle-cell anaemia
    (d)   iron deficiency anaemia
    (e)   macrocytosis.

7-17   Vitamin B_{12} deficiency can cause abnormalities apart from those of the blood. These include:

    (a)   peripheral neuropathy
    (b)   proximal myopathy
    (c)   optic atrophy
    (d)   subacute combined degeneration of the spinal cord
    (e)   hepatic failure.

7-18   There are many causes of splenomegaly. It might even be said by medical students that there are too many causes. The following are common causes of mild splenomegaly:

    (a)   infective endocarditis
    (b)   systemic lupus erythematosus
    (c)   Cushing's disease
    (d)   infectious mononucleosis
    (e)   antibiotic sensitivity.

7-19   A patient with pancytopenia may have:

    (a)   anaemia
    (b)   a raised platelet count
    (c)   a reduced neutrophil count
    (d)   an increased susceptibility to infection
    (e)   some form of underlying malignancy as the cause.

7-20   The following may occur in patients with acute leukaemia:

    (a)   tonsillar enlargement
    (b)   nerve palsy due to spinal root involvement
    (c)   bony tenderness
    (d)   splenic atrophy
    (e)   thrombocytosis.

7-21 Some patients with polycythaemia have increased erythropoietin levels. Erythropoietin may also be increased in the following conditions:

    (a) chronic renal failure
    (b) chronic hypoxia
    (c) acyanotic congenital heart disease
    (d) chronic hepatocellular carcinoma
    (e) erythropoietin tumours.

7-22 Patients with multiple myeloma may have signs of renal impairment. Renal impairment may occur in multiple myeloma for which of the following reasons?

    (a) hypercalcaemia
    (b) uric acid nephropathy
    (c) plasma cell infiltration
    (d) secondary amyloidosis
    (e) secondary to anaemia.

Chapter 8

The Rheumatological System

It has long been an axiom of mine that the little things are infinitely the most important. — Sherlock Holmes

(Sir Arthur Conan Doyle 1859–1930)

8-1 Patients who complain of joint pain but have no joint swelling:

(a) are said to have arthralgia
because
(b) the diagnosis of arthritis requires the presence of swelling as well as pain.

8-2 The presence of morning stiffness is an important symptom of joint disease:

(a) patients with morning stiffness are more likely to have inflammatory arthritis than osteoarthritis
(b) the length of time the stiffness lasts each day is a guide to severity
(c) the presence of morning stiffness is diagnostic of rheumatoid arthritis
(d) morning stiffness affects only the small joints in the hands and feet
(e) the presence of morning stiffness is an indication for the use of steroids in the treatment of arthritis.

8-3 Monoarthritis is inflammation of a single joint:

(a) sudden onset of monoarthritis without an obvious precipitating cause is characteristic of rheumatoid arthritis
(b) monoarthritis is only rarely due to infection
(c) monoarthritis can be a manifestation of gout
(d) patients should be asked about the possibility of trauma as the cause of their condition
(e) pseudogout does not cause monoarthritis.

8-4 Polyarthritis means the inflammation of a number of joints:

(a) the presence of polyarthritis always means that destructive changes will occur in the joints
(b) polyarthritis may sometimes be secondary to viral infection
(c) polyarthritis is never due to infection
(d) the diagnosis of rheumatoid arthritis in a patient presenting with polyarthritis can always be made on clinical examination
(e) other connective tissue disease such as lupus erythematosus may present with polyarthritis.

8-5 Certain patterns of polyarthritis may suggest the underlying diagnosis:

(a) rheumatoid arthritis is usually symmetrical and often affects the hands, particularly the proximal interphalangeal, metacarpophalangeal and wrist joints
(b) ankylosing spondylitis always involves the sacroiliac joints first
(c) psoriatic arthritis may affect the terminal interphalangeal joints
(d) psoriatic arthritis can occasionally present as seronegative arthritis with a rheumatoid arthritis pattern
(e) Reiter's syndrome may affect the ankles and joints of the feet early.

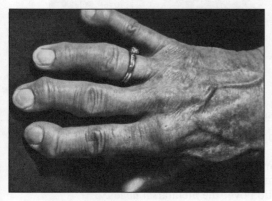

Photograph 8.1

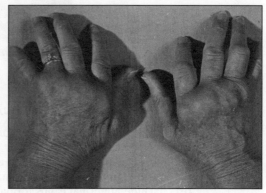

Photograph 8.2

8-6 The patient in Photograph 8.1:

(a) has changes characteristic of rheumatoid arthritis
(b) has changes suggestive of psoriatic arthritis
(c) has prominent Bouchard's nodes over the proximal and distal interphalangeal joints
(d) has changes characteristic of osteoarthritis
(e) has typical psoriatic nail changes.

8-7 Patients with Raynaud's phenomenon:

(a) tend not to like cold weather
(b) are more often women than men when the condition is idiopathic
(c) can have a condition made worse by certain drugs including beta-blockers
(d) may have the condition secondary to rheumatoid arthritis
(e) may have the condition secondary to renal failure.

8-8 The joint deformities present in the patient in Photograph 8.2 are:

(a) characteristic of rheumatoid arthritis
(b) subluxation of the metacarpophalangeal joints
(c) Z deformity of the thumbs
(d) Boutonniére deformity
(e) marked pannus formation over the wrists.

Photograph 8.3

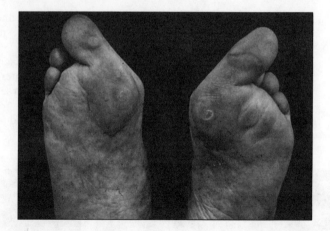

8-9   Changes in the patient's feet in Photograph 8.3:

    (a)   can be explained by the prolonged wearing of ill-fitting shoes
    (b)   include crowding of the toes
    (c)   are suggestive of rheumatoid arthritis
    (d)   include probable bunion formation
    (e)   include abnormal callus formation over the metatarsal heads.

Photograph 8.4

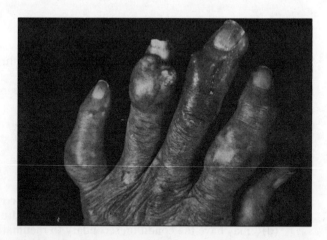

8-10   The deformities in the patient's hands in Photograph 8.4 suggest:

    (a)   active rheumatoid arthritis
    (b)   repeated trauma
    (c)   the presence of gout
    (d)   the presence of urate crystals
    (e)   the likely presence of psoriasis.

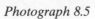
Photograph 8.5

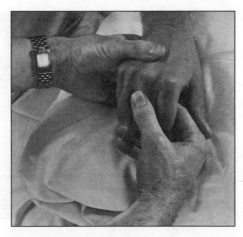

8-11 Examining the hands in the way shown in Photograph 8.5:

(a)   will usually cause pain and should be avoided
(b)   is a way of testing for abnormal movement at the metacarpophalangeal joint
(c)   will reveal abnormal signs in patients with rheumatoid arthritis in many cases
(d)   may also be a way of feeling for tendon crepitus in patients with rheumatoid arthritis
(e)   is not usually necessary on routine examination of the joints.

8-12 The patient in Photograph 8.6:

(a)   is unfortunate enough to have both rheumatoid arthritis and hyperlipidaemia
       because
(b)   tendon   xanthomata   are present at the elbows.

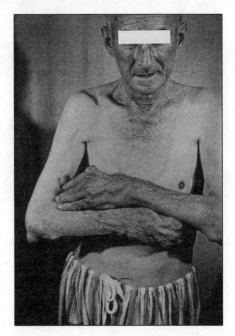

Photograph 8.6

Photograph 8.7

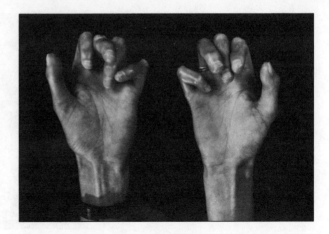

8-13 The patient in Photograph 8.7:

    (a)   has typical fixed flexion deformity from rheumatoid arthritis
    (b)   may well have difficulty swallowing
    (c)   is likely to have tethered skin on the dorsum of the hands
    (d)   is likely to have difficulty opening the mouth widely
    (e)   is very likely to have chronic liver disease.

8-14 In the examination of the hip joint:

    (a)   one should begin with inspection of the joint
    (b)   joint tenderness may be felt distal to the midpoint of the inguinal ligament
    (c)   it is not possible to test rotation
    (d)   abduction is usually possible to about 50 degrees
    (e)   adduction is rarely possible to more than 30 degrees.

8-15 On examination of the knee joint:

    (a)   one should test for collateral ligament movement
    (b)   cruciate ligaments are tested by attempting anterior and posterior movements of the leg on the knee joint
    (c)   flexion of the knee joint is usually possible to 135 degrees
    (d)   synovial swelling around the knee may be felt medial to the patella and in the joint suprapatellar extension
    (e)   quadriceps hypertrophy often occurs with arthritis of the knee joint.

8-16 A patient who has a toe that looks like a sausage (dactylitis):

    (a)   should be examined for the presence of a rash on the penis
    (b)   are likely to be rheumatoid factor positive
    (c)   may have pitting of the toe nails
    (d)   may have a typical psoriaform rash
    (e)   may have similar changes in a finger.

8-17   When the normal foot is examined:

    (a)   dorsiflexion at the talar (ankle) joint is normally possible to over 30 degrees

    (b)   plantar flexion of the same joint is normally only possible to 20 degrees

    (c)   movement at the subtalar joint includes inversion, eversion and flexion

    (d)   tenderness on movement of the subtalar joint is more important than the range of movement

    (e)   tenderness of the metatarsophalangeal joints is best assessed by compressing the first and fifth metatarsals.

8-18   Tenderness over the inferior aspect of the heel:

    (a)   may occur in the seronegative spondyloarthropathies
        because

    (b)   plantar fasciitis occurs in these conditions.

8-19   The general inspection of a patient with rheumatoid arthritis:

    (a)   may reveal a Cushingoid appearance
        because

    (b)   Cushing's disease is commonly associated with rheumatoid arthritis.

8-20   Examination of the eyes is important in patients suspected of suffering from rheumatoid arthritis. Abnormalities that may be found include:

    (a)   dryness due to Sjögren's syndrome

    (b)   the presence of a rheumatoid nodule in the sclera (episcleritis)

    (c)   iritis

    (d)   conjunctivitis

    (e)   conjunctival pallor indicating anaemia.

8-21   Examination of the heart is important in patients with rheumatoid arthritis. The following findings associated with the condition may be present:

    (a)   a pericardial rub

    (b)   dilated cardiomyopathy

    (c)   aortic regurgitation

    (d)   a fourth heart sound (S4)

    (e)   atrial fibrillation.

8-22   Abnormalities of the knees in patients with rheumatoid arthritis include:

    (a)   the presence of Baker's cysts in the popliteal fossae

    (b)   synovial effusions

    (c)   quadriceps wasting

    (d)   ligamentous instability

    (e)   the presence of rheumatoid nodules.

8-23   Footdrop:

    (a)   may complicate rheumatoid arthritis
          because
    (b)   lumbar disc disease is common.

8-24   Which of the following is *not* one of the seronegative spondyloarthropathies (choose the one best answer)?

    (a)   Ankylosing spondylitis
    (b)   Psoriatic arthritis
    (c)   Reiter's disease
    (d)   Mixed connective tissue disease
    (e)   Enteropathic arthritis.

8-25   Reiter's syndrome usually causes asymmetrical arthritis involving the large joints. The following abnormalities may be found:

    (a)   circinate balanitis
    (b)   conjunctivitis
    (c)   very painful mouth ulcers
    (d)   occasional involvement of the wrists
    (e)   rheumatoid nodules.

8-26   Enteropathic arthritis is an uncommon condition:

    (a)   it is usually associated with ulcerative colitis but not Crohn's disease
    (b)   one form involves peripheral joints
    (c)   peripheral joint involvement is usually symmetrical
    (d)   another form is very similar to ankylosing spondylitis
    (e)   joint deformity is common.

8-27   Gouty tophi can affect a number of parts of the body. The area least likely to be involved is (choose the one best answer):

    (a)   the Achilles tendon
    (b)   the infrapatellar tendon
    (c)   the extensor surface of the fingers
    (d)   the helix of the ear
    (e)   the costochondral junctions.

8-28   Systemic lupus erythematosus (SLE) is a chronic inflammatory disease which affects many parts of the body. Which of the following is *least likely* to be related to the disease (choose the one best answer):

    (a)   psychosis
    (b)   photosensitivity rashes
    (c)   Raynaud's phenomenon
    (d)   the presence of rheumatoid nodules
    (e)   synovitis involving the proximal metacarpophalangeal joints.

8-29   Hair changes should be looked for in patients with SLE. The common abnormalities of the hair include:

(a)   short broken hairs above the forehead
(b)   alopecia (hair loss)
(c)   changes in hair appearance so that it looks greasy
(d)   abnormal hair growth on the face
(e)   hair changes similar to those in hypothyroidism.

8-30   SLE may cause eyes signs. The *least likely* abnormality to be found is (choose the one best answer):

(a)   conjunctival pallor
(b)   jaundice
(c)   the presence of cytoid bodies
(d)   lens dislocation
(e)   changes similar to those in Sjögren's syndrome.

8-31   Scleroderma or progressive systemic sclerosis is a connective tissue disease characterised by cutaneous fibrosis. The general inspection of the patient with scleroderma may reveal the following changes:

(a)   weight gain and a Cushingoid appearance
(b)   non-pitting oedema of the hands
(c)   thickening and induration of the skin of the hands and forearms
(d)   the presence of calcific deposits in the subcutaneous tissues of the fingers (calcinosis)
(e)   Raynaud's phenomenon which is, however, very rare.

8-32   Rheumatic fever is an uncommon condition in developed countries today. The diagnosis is quite difficult and depends on the presence of major and minor criteria. The following are major criteria for the diagnosis of rheumatic fever:

(a)   polyarthritis
(b)   the presence of a red throat
(c)   the presence of a new cardiac murmur
(d)   subcutaneous nodules
(e)   the presence of chorea.

Chapter 9

The Endocrine System

*What we think and feel and are is to a great extent determined
by the state of our ductless glands and our viscera*

Aldous Huxley (1894–1964)

9-1 Endocrinologists claim endocrinology is the most interesting medical speciality because endocrine disorders can affect many different parts of the body. Which one of the following is most likely to be a manifestation of endocrine disease (choose the one best answer)?

(a) Changes in body hair distribution
(b) Tall stature
(c) Headache
(d) Male baldness
(e) Increased tendency to sweat.

9-2 Which of the following disorders can be associated with weight gain?

(a) Hypothyroidism
(b) Greed
(c) Cushing's syndrome
(d) Uncontrolled diabetes mellitus
(e) Malignancy.

9-3 The acral changes that occur in acromegaly tend to be of very gradual onset. They may be missed by both doctors and relatives who see the patient regularly. Changes in the clinical appearance associated with acromegaly include:

(a) coarse facial features
(b) a large tongue
(c) an increase in head size
(d) increased pitch in the voice
(e) enlargement of the hands and feet.

9-4 Diabetes mellitus may be diagnosed by routine blood sugar estimation. Some patients present without symptoms. Common presentations can include all of the following *except* (choose the one best answer):

(a) decreased appetite always
(b) blurred vision
(c) weakness
(d) thrush
(e) skin infections.

9-5   Lethargy is a very common presenting symptom, but an endocrine cause is uncommon. The following endocrine diseases, however, can produce lethargy:

(a)   thyrotoxicosis
(b)   diabetes mellitus
(c)   adrenal failure
(d)   phaeochromocytoma
(e)   hyperinsulinaemia.

9-6   Patients with endocrine disorders may present to a dermatologist because of skin changes. Which one of the following skin changes is *least likely* to be associated with an endocrine disorder (choose the one best answer):

(a)   appearance of skin tags
(b)   increased pigmentation
(c)   flushing of the face and neck
(d)   scattered areas of skin atrophy
(e)   unpleasant black discoloration in the axillae.

9-7   Causes of short stature include:

(a)   childhood hypothyroidism
(b)   childhood pituitary failure
(c)   short parents
(d)   Klinefelter's syndrome
(e)   primary adrenal failure.

9-8   The following is the most likely cause of male impotence (choose the one best answer):

(a)   psychological distress
(b)   diabetes mellitus
(c)   hypogonadism
(d)   hyperprolactinaemia
(e)   haemochromatosis.

9-9   Primary amenorrhoea:

(a)   is defined as failure to begin menstruation by the age of 15 years
(b)   is most commonly caused by excess androgen production
(c)   can be caused by chronic renal failure
(d)   can be caused by malnutrition
(e)   can sometimes be the result of psychiatric disease.

9-10   Polyuria can be caused by a number of endocrine and other disorders. A patient who complains of this symptom:

(a)   needs to be carefully questioned so that urinary frequency can be distinguished from polyuria
(b)   by definition passes more than three litres of urine a day
(c)   may have diabetes mellitus but not diabetes insipidus
(d)   may drink too much water
(e)   can be reassured that he or she does not suffer from renal failure.

9-11   Many clues to endocrine disease can be obtained when a careful history is taken from the patient. The following feature of the patient history is *least likely* to indicate a significant endocrine abnormality (choose the one best answer):

(a)   the recent birth of a very large baby
(b)   diagnosis of carcinoma of the lung
(c)   history of skin and foot infections
(d)   previous surgery on the neck
(e)   unexplained weight gain.

9-12   Diabetes mellitus is a chronic disease and patients should be well informed about their condition. A patient should reasonably be expected to:

(a)   understand the difference between human and animal insulins
(b)   know his or her current insulin dose
(c)   be familiar with the symptoms of hypoglycaemia
(d)   be able to test the urine for sugar but *not* the blood for sugar
(e)   understand the principles of treatment of diabetic ketoacidosis.

9-13   A patient with established hypoadrenalism should be aware of some of the problems associated with this condition. It is reasonable to expect such a patient to:

(a)   adjust his or her steroid dose at times of mental stress
(b)   know the need to inform his or her doctor of the condition before any surgical operation is undertaken
(c)   know how to adjust the timing of the steroid doses during daily activities
(d)   have some idea of the basis of the condition and the reason for treatment
(e)   be able to test the blood for cortisol levels.

9-14   Which of the following statements is correct concerning thyroid examination?

(a)   the normal thyroid gland is never palpable
(b)   The normal gland can often be detected extending slightly into the chest
(c)   An enlarged thyroid gland (goitre) can often be diagnosed on inspection
(d)   As the patient sips a glass of water, the gland can be felt to move down slightly during swallowing
(e)   Enlarged thyroids are almost always tender.

9-15   Causes of a mass in the neck include:

(a)   a thyroglossal cyst
(b)   lymphoma
(c)   a normal carotid artery
(d)   a trachea that is unusually anteriorly placed
(e)   a lymph node.

9-16   The patient in Photograph 9.1 has lost weight recently. The most likely cause is (choose the one best answer):

- (a)   adrenal failure
- (b)   starvation
- (c)   carcinoma of the colon
- (d)   thyrotoxicosis
- (e)   panhypopituitarism.

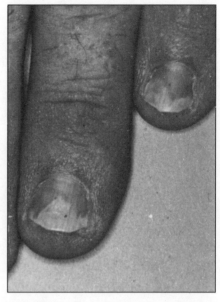

Photograph 9.1

9-17   The patient in Photograph 9.2 is lethargic. The examination is likely to reveal:

- (a)   dry skin
- (b)   increased reflexes
- (c)   tachycardia
- (d)   spade-like hands
- (e)   croaking, slow speech

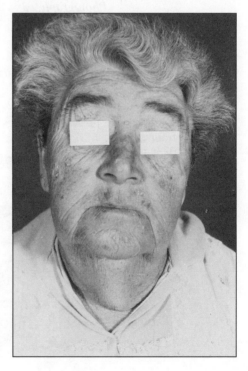

Photograph 9.2

9-18   The patient in Photograph 9.3 does not have any symptoms. Examination, however, may well reveal:

    (a)   macroglossia
    (b)   proximal muscle weakness
    (c)   bitemporal hemianopia
    (d)   hands that will not fit into large surgical gloves
    (e)   axillary hair loss.

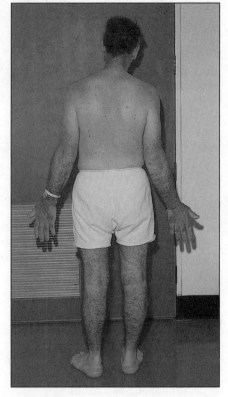

Photograph 9.3

9-19   Possible causes of the man's problem in Photograph 9.4 include:

    (a)   a testicular tumour
    (b)   hepatic failure
    (c)   use of certain prescription drugs
    (d)   trauma
    (e)   diabetes mellitus.

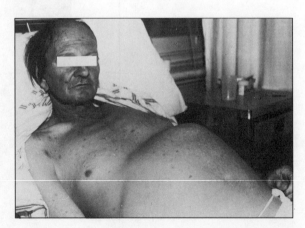

Photograph 9.4

Photograph 9.5

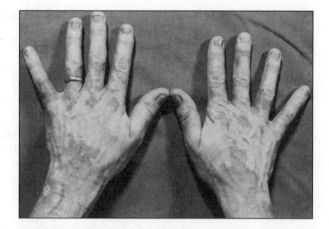

9-20 The hands of the patient in Photograph 9.5:

- (a) show the typical hyperpigmentation of primary hypoadrenalism
- (b) may be associated with autoimmune adrenal failure
- (c) are not usually associated with pigmentary changes elsewhere in the body
- (d) can be associated with pernicious anaemia
- (e) may be found in patients with thyroid disease.

Photograph 9.6

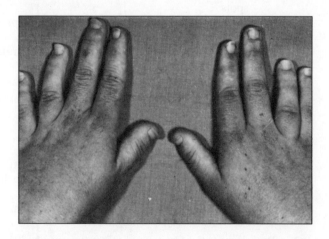

9-21 The patient in Photograph 9.6 has problems with recurrent attacks of tetany. He:

- (a) is likely to have low levels of parathyroid hormone
- (b) is likely to have a positive Trousseau's sign
- (c) may show a facial muscle twitch if the facial nerve is tapped (Chvostek's sign)
- (d) may have changes in the toes to match his hands
- (e) is likely to be tall and thin.

9-22   Woman who are hairier than they feel they should be:

(a)   will almost always have an endocrine abnormality
(b)   should be examined for signs of virilisation
(c)   can always be reassured this is a normal variant
(d)   may have polycystic ovaries
(e)   should be asked about any drugs they are taking.

9-23   Down's syndrome is a relatively common abnormality involving trisomy of chromosome 21. There are a number of characteristic features. These include:

(a)   short broad hands
(b)   reduced joint flexibility
(c)   oblique orbital fissures
(d)   a flat low palate
(e)   an increased risk of atrial and ventricular septal defect.

9-24   One of the important complications of diabetes mellitus involves changes in the retina:

(a)   proliferative retinal changes are less likely to interfere with vision than non-proliferative ones
(b)   minor changes including dot haemorrhages are present in all diabetics if the retinas are examined carefully enough
(c)   laser scars may be present in the retina; these may appear as small dark spots
(d)   the new vessel formation characteristic of proliferative change may improve retinal function
(e)   hard exudates are considered a non-proliferative change.

9-25   Queen Victoria's surgeon, Sir James Paget, has two diseases named after him. Osteitis deformans or Paget's disease of bone is one of them. Paget's disease of bone:

(a)   is due to reduced osteoclast activity
(b)   is likely to be of bacterial origin
(c)   may cause pronounced lower limb deformity
(d)   may be responsible for the presence of bronchial breath sounds over the skull
(e)   may occasionally be complicated by sarcoma.

9-26   Paget's disease of bone may affect the eyes and the cranial nerves. In Paget's disease of bone:

(a)   angioid streaks may be present in the fundi
(b)   deafness may occur because of eighth nerve compression or involvement of the ossicles
(c)   anosmia is usually associated
(d)   the lower cranial nerves may be affected because of bony overgrowth of the foramina
(e)   only men are affected.

9-27 Pigment changes:

(a) occur in Addison's disease
because
(b) adrenocorticotrophic hormone (ACTH) has melanocyte stimulating activity.

9-28 Palpation of the abdomen of patients with suspected Cushing's syndrome:

(a) is useful
because
(b) large adrenal carcinomas are a common cause of the condition.

9-29 Patients with acromegaly:

(a) may have enlarged testes
because
(b) of the effects of growth hormone.

Chapter 10

The Nervous System

Now, what I want is facts ... facts alone are wanted in life.

Hard Times — Charles Dickens (1812–1870)

10-1   A 47-year-old woman comes to her doctor with a 15-year history of recurrent headaches. The headache is non-throbbing, present bilaterally over the top of the head and is not associated with photophobia, blurring of vision, rhinorrhoea, fever or vomiting. The most likely cause of the headache is (choose the one best answer):

   (a)   tension headache
   (b)   classic migraine
   (c)   cluster headache
   (d)   subarachnoid haemorrhage
   (e)   brain tumour.

10-2   Neck stiffness:

   (a)   strongly suggests a higher centre disorder
   (b)   must be looked for in any febrile patient
   (c)   indicates an upper motor neurone lesion
   (d)   is a sign of alcoholism
   (e)   indicates raised intracranial pressure.

10-3   Match the following speech patterns with the type of dysphasia:

   (a)   disorganised fluent speech but difficulty understanding commands
   (b)   slurred speech
   (c)   normal speech but unable to name objects

   1.   nominal dysphasia
   2.   dysarthria
   3.   receptive (Wernicke's) dysphasia
   4.   expressive (Broca's) dysphasia
   5.   dysphonia

10-4   With regard to the visual field examination, which of the following are true?

   (a)   Parietal lobe lesions produce a bitemporal hemianopia
   (b)   Papilloedema can cause peripheral constriction of visual fields (but not true tunnel vision)
   (c)   A tumour in the temporal lobe can produce a homonymous hemianopia
   (d)   Optic nerve disease can cause loss of vision in one eye
   (e)   The blind spot can be mapped.

10-5   Causes of fundal haemorrhages seen on fundoscopy include:

  (a) diabetes mellitus
  (b) subarachnoid haemorrhage
  (c) hypertension
  (d) retinitis pigmentosa
  (e) bleeding diathesis.

10-6   A patient presents with a history of being blind in the left eye since birth. On examination, you find that on repeatedly moving your torch from the normal eye to the eye with zero visual acuity, the pupil, instead of constricting normally to light, paradoxically dilates in the affected eye. Of the following statements, which are correct:

  (a) this sign indicates that the patient is hysterical and really can see with the left eye
  (b) this sign suggests left optic atrophy
  (c) this is called an Argyll-Robertson pupil and results from syphilis
  (d) this is called the Marcus Gunn phenomenon *– paradoxical dil?*
  (e) this is a useful test of accommodation.

10-7   Nystagmus can be caused by: *vect*

  (a) alcohol
  (b) drugs such as phenytoin
  (c) brainstem lesions
  (d) vestibular lesions
  (e) decreased macular vision.

10-8   The corneal reflex:

  (a) tests cerebellar function
  (b) tests macular vision
  (c) tests cranial nerve VIII function
  (d) tests cranial nerves V and VII function
  (e) is not a useful test.

10-9   An upper motor neurone facial palsy produces:

  (a) Bell's palsy
  (b) weak forehead muscles on testing the affected side
  (c) drooping of the corner of the mouth
  (d) absence of Bell's phenomenon (which is upward eyeball movement and incomplete eyelid closure)
  (e) loss of facial sensation on the affected side.

10-10   A patient complaining of increasing deafness is tested as follows. A vibrating 256 hertz tuning fork is placed on the mastoid process and when the sound can no longer be heard by the patient it is placed in line with the external ear. The patient reports that he can now hear the vibrating sound again. This result suggests (choose the one best answer):

(a)   nerve deafness
(b)   conduction deafness
(c)   no real deafness
(d)   otitis media
(e)   wax in the ear.

10-11   Absence of the gag reflex may indicate:

(a)   a lower motor neurone IX nerve palsy
(b)   a lower motor neurone XI nerve palsy
(c)   an upper motor neurone VII nerve palsy
(d)   a lower motor neurone V nerve palsy
(e)   an upper motor neurone XII nerve palsy.

Photograph 10.1

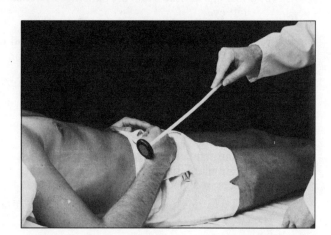

10-12   In Photograph 10.1, the examiner:

(a)   is eliciting the brachioradialis jerk
(b)   is testing the C5 and C6 segmental innervation
(c)   will normally expect extension of the elbow
(d)   is testing the C8 segmental innervation
(e)   is testing for finger jerks.

10-13   Fasciculations are irregular non-rhythmical contractions of muscle fascicles. Fasciculations:

(a)   indicate that the diagnosis is definitely motor neurone disease
(b)   occur in Horner's syndrome
(c)   are usually benign if there is no weakness or wasting of the muscles
(d)   are always best elicited by tapping over the muscle
(e)   can occur in thyrotoxicosis.

Photograph 10.2

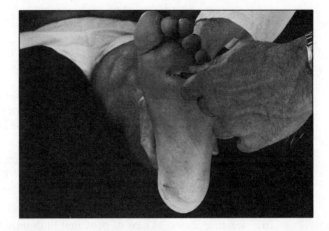

10-14   In Photograph 10.2, the examiner:

   (a)   should stroke up the lateral aspect of the sole and then curve inwards

   (b)   should expect flexion of the big toe in an adult to occur normally

   (c)   may observe bilateral upgoing toes in comatose patients

   (d)   should observe bilateral upgoing toes in paraplegia

   (e)   should observe a unilateral upgoing toe in hemiplegia on the affected side of the body.

10-15   During your neurological examination of a middle-aged man, you ask the patient to hold out his arms extended and close his eyes. You observe downward drifting of his right arm from the neutral position. You interpret this correctly as evidence that:

   (a)   he may have right-sided upper motor neurone weakness from a stroke

   (b)   he has a right-sided tremor

   (c)   he may have a lesion in the left cerebellar hemisphere

   (d)   he still has normal joint position sense

   (e)   he has fasciculations.

10-16   As a patient walks into your room in the outpatients department, you notice that he has an abnormal gait. Which of the following statements are correct?

   (a)   If the foot is plantar flexed and the leg is swung in a lateral arc this suggests footdrop from a common peroneal nerve palsy

   (b)   If the gait is shuffling and the patient has difficulty stopping, he may have Parkinson's disease

   (c)   A waddling gait occurs in hemiplegic patients

   (d)   A clumsy slapping down of the feet occurs in Vitamin B_{12} deficiency

   (e)   If the feet appear to be glued to the floor he may have a tumour of the frontal lobe of the brain.

10-17   In hemisection of the thoracic spinal cord, you are likely to find on examination:

    (a)   weakness and spasticity below the level of the lesion on the same side
    (b)   loss of vibration and proprioception below the lesion on the opposite side
    (c)   loss of pain and temperature below the lesion on the same side
    (d)   lower motor neurone signs above the level of the lesion on the same side
    (e)   unilateral pain and temperature loss on the face.

10-18   A 45-year-old balding man shakes your hand on meeting you in the office, but is unable to let go of your hand immediately. Which of the following signs would you look for in this man?

    (a)   partial ptosis
    (b)   wasting and weakness of proximal limb muscles
    (c)   testicular atrophy
    (d)   senile cataracts and subcapsular deposits
    (e)   sugar in the urine.

10-19   With an ulnar nerve lesion at the wrist:

    (a)   partial clawing of the hand may occur
    (b)   sensory loss occurs over the thumb
    (c)   wrist drop does *not* occur
    (d)   the thumb can abduct normally
    (e)   wasting of the small hand muscles occurs.

10-20   Causes of tremor include:

    (a)   Parkinson's disease
    (b)   thyrotoxicosis
    (c)   chorea
    (d)   dystonia
    (e)   cerebellar disease.

10-21   In Figure 10.3, a lesion at the site marked 5 would produce:

    (a)   homonymous hemianopia
    (b)   central scotomata
    (c)   bitemporal hemianopia
    (d)   unilateral field loss
    (e)   tunnel vision.

10-22   In Figure 10.3, a lesion at the site marked 6 would produce:

    (a)   homonymous hemianopia
    (b)   central scotomata
    (c)   bitemporal hemianopia
    (d)   unilateral field loss
    (e)   tunnel vision.

Figure 10.3

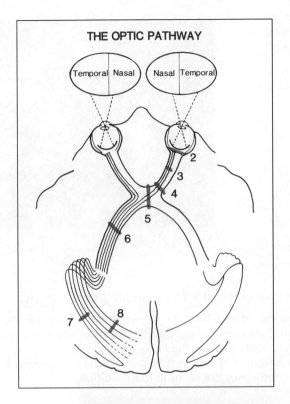

THE OPTIC PATHWAY

Photograph 10.4

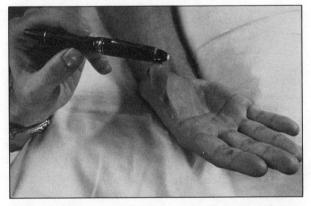

10-23 The patient performs the pen-touching test in Photograph 10.4 as shown as part of the upper limb examination. You should conclude:

   (a)   there is a median nerve palsy at the wrist
   (b)   there is likely to be sensory loss over the palmar aspect of the thumb, index and middle fingers
   (c)   there is an ulnar nerve palsy
   (d)   the abductor pollicis brevis is intact
   (e)   there is a radial nerve palsy.

Photograph 10.5

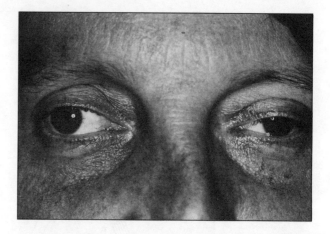

10-24 Look at Photograph 10.5. The following are correct:

    (a)   you should look for pain and temperature loss over the face and limbs
    (b)   you should feel for increased sweating over the affected eyebrow
    (c)   myasthenia gravis is the likely diagnosis
    (d)   a respiratory system examination should be performed
    (e)   exophthalmos can occur in this condition.

10-25 Regarding the dermatomes, as a rough rule of the thumb, the following are correct:

    (a)   S3, S4 and S5 supply the anus
    (b)   C5 supplies the shoulder tip
    (c)   L2 supplies the upper thigh
    (d)   C8 supplies the little finger
    (e)   S1 supplies the heel.

10-26 On testing tone at the wrists and elbows during an upper limb neurological examination, you find that tone is increased. This could be due to:

    (a)   a peripheral nerve lesion
    (b)   Parkinson's syndrome
    (c)   chorea
    (d)   an upper motor neurone lesion
    (e)   mononeuritis multiplex.

10-27 Whilst examining a 30-year-old woman with known long-standing Crohn's disease of the terminal ileum, you observe normal muscle bulk but detect weakness of hip, knee and ankle dorsiflexion, and weak hip abduction. Tone is also increased at the knees and ankles, with clonus. In addition, you find that the knee and ankle reflexes in both legs are absent but there is an extensor plantar response. On testing sensation, vibration and joint position sense are lost in both legs, but pain sensation is normal. There are no cerebellar signs present. You conclude that:

(a) she may have subacute combined degeneration of the spinal cord
(b) she may be vitamin B$_{12}$ deficient
(c) she may have had a stroke
(d) she may have motor neurone disease
(e) she most likely has Friedreich's ataxia.

10-28 When examining for cerebellar signs, you should:

(a) look for nystagmus
(b) determine if speech is jerky, explosive and loud
(c) test for hypotonia and pendular reflexes in the limbs
(d) look for intention tremor and past-pointing with the finger-nose test
(e) test for an ataxic gait.

10-29 In the comatose patient, doll's eye testing is useful. The following is/are correct:

(a) doll's eye testing is performed by rolling the head gently from side to side with the eyelids opened by the examiner
(b) the eyes move with the head if the brainstem is intact
(c) if the eyes maintain their fixation, this suggests a brainstem lesion
(d) doll's eyes are tonic deviation of both eyes to one side
(e) the cranial nerves cannot be assessed in coma.

10-30 In a comatose patient:

(a) you must look for evidence of hypoglycaemia
    because
(b) giving intravenous glucose can save the life of a comatose patient with hypoglycaemia.

10-31 In which of the following are the associated features correctly linked to the underlying cause?

(a) Trigeminal sensory loss: trigeminal neuralgia
(b) Onset in old age: temporal arteritis
(c) Worse when lying down: raised intracranial pressure
(d) Oculomotor palsy: posterior communicating artery aneurysm
(e) Female predominance: cluster headache.

10-32 Which of the following are well recognised causes of ataxia and nystagmus?

(a) Phenytoin toxicity
(b) Middle cerebral artery thrombosis
(c) Posterior fossa tumour
(d) Alcoholic brain damage
(e) Multiple sclerosis.

10-33   The following statements are true of patients with Parkinson's disease:

(a)   resting tremor is a common presenting feature
(b)   upper motor neurone signs are often found in the arms
(c)   at post-mortem examination, a characteristic finding is depigmentation of the substantia nigra
(d)   the disease is always idiopathic in aetiology
(e)   frequent falls are a common problem.

10-34   A 61-year-old woman has suffered several recent episodes of transient aphasia and right arm weakness. The following statements concerning her are true:

(a)   examination of the left fundus may help with the diagnosis
(b)   multiple sclerosis is a likely cause
(c)   one should listen for carotid bruits
(d)   a brain tumour is the most likely cause
(e)   examining the cardiovascular system is *not* likely to be of much help.

10-35   Typical features of Alzheimer's disease include:

(a)   early development of urinary incontinence
(b)   the sudden onset of symptoms
(c)   a rapid stepwise progression of symptoms
(d)   disturbance of visuo-spatial skills
(e)   disturbance of language/dysphasia.

10-36   A 45-year-old man presents with a painless left foot drop, which developed over two days. On examination there is weakness of toe extension and eversion of the ankle. Sensation is impaired over the lateral aspect of the dorsum of the foot. The reflexes are normal. The following diagnosis is most likely with these symptoms and signs (choose the one best answer):

(a)   a left common peroneal nerve lesion
(b)   amyotrophic lateral sclerosis
(c)   a lacunar stroke involving the left internal capsule
(d)   an L3 nerve root compression due to an intervertebral disc herniation
(e)   Horner' syndrome.

10-37   As part of a neurological examination two patients were asked to copy the upper drawings (Figure 10.6). The first copied the first two. From these attempts at copying the examiner could reasonably conclude that:

(a)   the patient might also have difficulty putting on an inside-out cardigan
(b)   the patient has a dominant parietal lesion
(c)   the patient is left handed
(d)   visual inattention may be present
(e)   the patient may have agraphaesthesia.

Figure 10.6

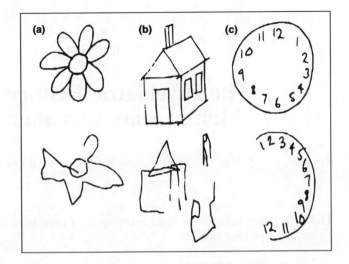

10-38   The second patient attempted to copy drawing C (Figure 10.6). This patient:

  (a)   is more likely to have a non-dominant than a dominant parietal lesion
  (b)   is suffering from spatial neglect
  (c)   is likely to have anosmia
  (d)   is unlikely to have any difficulty with the cardigan
  (e)   will probably have dysphasia.

10-39   The following are features of papilloedema rather than of papillitis:

  (a)   normal visual acuity
  (b)   pain on eye movement
  (c)   colour vision (especially red vision) affected early
  (d)   bilateral occurrence
  (e)   sudden onset.

10-40   The following are features of a third nerve palsy:

  (a)   a constricted pupil
  (b)   reduced sweating on the forehead on the affected side
  (c)   ptosis
  (d)   a dilated pupil which is reactive to direct light but not to accommodation
  (e)   divergent visual axes.

Chapter 11

The Psychiatric History and Mental State Examination

Most of the time we think we're sick it's all in the mind

Thomas Wolfe (1900–1938)

11-1 The first thing to do when carrying out a psychiatric interview is to (choose the one best answer):

(a) test orientation
(b) establish rapport
(c) make a diagnosis
(d) make a biopsychosocial formulation
(e) give advice.

11-2 Perceptual disturbances include all the following except (choose the one best answer):

(a) hallucinations
(b) hypnagogic experiences
(c) echolalia
(d) depersonalisation
(e) derealisation.

11-3 Asking patients what they would do if they found someone else's mail lying in the street is an example of a test of (choose the one best answer):

(a) intelligence
(b) abstract thinking
(c) insight
(d) judgment
(e) cognition.

11-4 Methods to facilitate the development of rapport include all the following except (choose the one best answer):

(a) conducting a stress interview
(b) asking open-ended questions
(c) using the patient's words
(d) understanding the patient
(e) uncovering feelings.

11-5   The patient's vocabulary and fund of knowledge on a mental status examination are the best guides to:

(a)   intelligence
(b)   attention
(c)   memory and orientation
(d)   abstract thinking
(e)   judgment.

11-6   Assessing suicidal risk:

(a)   puts thoughts of suicide into the patient's mind
(b)   is best done by asking the patient if he or she has thought of attempting suicide
(c)   is essential for all depressed patients
(d)   should only be done indirectly
(e)   increases the risk of the patient attempting suicide.

11-7   Clouding of consciousness is a feature of:

(a)   schizophrenia
(b)   high levels of anxiety
(c)   delirium
(d)   dementia
(e)   sleep.

11-8   The mental state examination:

(a)   should be performed after the physical examination
(b)   can only be done by a psychiatrist
(c)   consists only of tests of memory
(d)   includes your observations of the patient throughout the interview
(e)   includes tests of cognitive functioning.

11-9   For each of the numbered statements below, select the one lettered word that is most closely associated with it.

1.   a normal human emotion
2.   a repetitive, irrational and resisted thought
3.   an irrational fear
4.   a sensory perception without a stimulus
5.   a false, fixed belief out of keeping with the patient's culture

(a)   hallucination
(b)   delusion
(c)   depression
(d)   obsession
(e)   phobia

Chapter 12

The Skin

Dermatology is the best speciality. The patient
never dies — and never gets well.

Anonymous

12-1   Certain skin diseases such as leprosy and syphilis:

(a)   can cause anaesthesia
because
(b)   they involve neurovascular bundles or nerves.

12-2   When the dermatological history is taken:

(a)   systemic symptoms such as fever, anorexia and weight loss must be asked about
because
(b)   a number of systemic diseases affect the skin.

12-3   When a skin lump is examined:

(a)   the diagnosis of a sebaceous cyst can be made with certainty if the lump is within the skin
(b)   if a mass arises from the subcutaneous tissue, the skin can always be moved freely over the top of it
(c)   a mass in a muscle or tendon will be less mobile when the muscle is contracted
(d)   a mass growing from a nerve may be associated with paraesthesiae in the distribution of that nerve when the area is pressed
(e)   a lump over bone will always be tender.

12-4   If a cutaneous mass contains fluid:

(a)   it may be fluctuant
(b)   it will always transilluminate
(c)   it is unlikely to be due to inflammation unless warmth and redness are present
(d)   if it is due to inflammation, the draining lymph nodes will always be palpable
(e)   it is unlikely to be a neurofibroma.

12-5 Pruritus means itchiness. Generalised pruritus may be due to:

- (a) cholestasis
- (b) chronic renal failure
- (c) Addison's disease
- (d) lymphoma
- (e) psychogenic factors.

12-6 Erythrosquamous eruptions are red and scaly. They are not always well demarcated, and they are sometimes itchy. The following statements are true:

- (a) itchy erythrosquamous lesions on the palms and soles suggest secondary syphilis
- (b) lichen planus may cause asymptomatic lesions in the same areas
- (c) intensely itchy, diffuse lesions may be due to nummular eczema
- (d) well demarcated scaly lesions on the extensor surfaces are typical of psoriasis
- (e) scattered lesions on the trunk may be caused by pityriasis rosea.

12-7 There are a number of blistering skin diseases; some of these represent dermatological emergencies, but are rare. Blistering or bullous eruptions:

- (a) may occur in viral illnesses such as herpes simplex
- (b) may occur in herpes zoster but in this condition they usually do not cross far over the midline of the body
- (c) may be widespread and itchy in patients with dermatitis herpetiformis
- (d) may occur in porphyria cutanea tarda
- (e) never leave scars.

12-8 Erythroderma:

- (a) may be a dermatological emergency
  because
- (b) exfoliation of large amounts of skin may occur with loss of fluid and electrolytes.

12-9 A pustular lesion:

- (a) is always due to infection
  because
- (b) it contains neutrophils.

12-10 Erythema nodosum is one of a group of diseases called the nodular vasculitides. Erythema nodosum:

- (a) is typically found anywhere on the body
- (b) can be associated with inflammatory bowel disease
- (c) may occur in patients with tuberculosis, but only if the condition is extrapulmonary
- (d) can occur in sarcoidosis
- (e) may represent a drug reaction; for example, to sulfonamides.

12-11   Patients with excessive sweating (more discreetly named hyperhidrosis) may present to a dermatologist. Possible causes of this condition include:

   (a)   hypothyroidism
   (b)   acromegaly
   (c)   hypoglycaemia
   (d)   autonomic dysfunction
   (e)   fever.

12-12   Ulcers of the skin which do not heal:

   (a)   should usually be biopsied
         because
   (b)   they frequently represent malignant skin tumours.

12-13   Patients at increased risk of malignant melanoma include:

   (a)   people living in the tropics
   (b)   Australian Aborigines
   (c)   those who have inherited increased skin pigmentation
   (d)   people with the dysplastic naevus syndrome
   (e)   people with numerous solar keratoses.

12-14   The following conditions may be diagnosed by an alert dermatologist on inspection of the skin:

   (a)   dermatomyositis
   (b)   rheumatic fever
   (c)   neurofibromatosis
   (d)   infective endocarditis
   (e)   recent oral steroid use.

Chapter 13

Infectious Diseases

Fever, the eternal reproach to the physicians.

John Milton (1608–1674)

13-1 Pyrexia (or fever) of unknown origin (PUO) is defined as fever of more than 38 degrees Celsius for more than three weeks' duration without an obvious cause. In these patients:

    (a)   the longer the duration of fever, the more likely an infection will eventually be found

    (b)   a rare disease is usually found to be the explanation

    (c)   in almost all cases the aetiology is never found

    (d)   neoplasia is the cause in about 30% of cases

    (e)   connective tissue disease is an explanation in some patients.

13-2 In patients with prolonged fever and a rash:

    (a)   a drug reaction should be considered

    (b)   bacterial infection such as syphilis may occasionally be the cause

    (c)   acute viral hepatitis can be the cause

    (d)   connective tissue disease such as systemic lupus erythematosus should be considered

    (e)   history of travel to the tropics should be sought.

13-3 In patients with prolonged fever:

    (a)   fungal infections are not likely to be the cause
        because

    (b)   they do not cause fever.

13-4 Examination of the abdomen may be helpful in patients with pyrexia of unknown origin. It is important to look for:

    (a)   the presence of a tender mass suggesting an abscess

    (b)   inguinal lymphadenopathy

    (c)   the presence of splenomegaly

    (d)   para-aortic nodes suggestive of typhoid

    (e)   a rectal mass.

13-5   When a patient who is human immunodeficiency virus (HIV) antibody positive is examined:

(a)   there may be generalised wasting

(b)   drug treatment may have resulted in increased pigmentation

(c)   herpes zoster is most likely to be found in very advanced cases of acquired immunodeficiency syndrome (AIDS)

(d)   acute HIV infection (the seroconversion illness) may be suspected if a maculopapular rash is present some weeks after a possible exposure to the virus

(e) . lesions of Kaposi's sarcoma may be present and are usually raised and not tender.

13-6   Examination of the mouth of a patient with HIV/AIDS may commonly reveal:

(a)   herpes simplex virus ulceration of the tongue

(b)   Kaposi's lesions on the palate

(c)   white hairy lesions on the tongue — hairy leukoplakia

(d)   macroglossia

(e)   periodontal disease.

Chapter 14

Final Quiz

Statistics will prove anything, even the truth.

Lord Moynihan

R-1 The following symptoms and signs suggest a diagnosis of myocarditis or pericarditis:

(a)   sharp chest pain which is worse on deep breathing
(b)   recent onset of dyspnoea of effort
(c)   irregular heart beat
(d)   cough
(e)   exertional chest tightness.

R-2 The following is/are recognised symptom(s) of gastro-oesophageal reflux disease:

(a)   chronic cough
(b)   lethargy from iron deficiency anaemia
(c)   haematemesis
(d)   hoarseness
(e)   dysphagia.

R-3 The following is/are documented opportunistic gastrointestinal pathogens and cause diarrhoea in patients with the acquired immunodeficiency syndrome (AIDS):

(a)   cytomegalovirus
(b)   echovirus
(c)   *Toxoplasma gondii*
(d)   microsporidium
(e)   cryptosporidium.

R-4 The following is/are useful for assessing the activity of the arthritis in patients with rheumatoid arthritis:

(a)   the number of swollen joints
(b)   IgM rheumatoid factor level
(c)   degree of anaemia
(d)   duration of morning stiffness
(e)   fever.

R-5   The following is/are recognised feature(s) in the first 24 hours of lobar pneumonia in an otherwise healthy person:

(a)   a swinging fever
(b)   a sore throat
(c)   nasal stuffiness
(d)   bronchial breathing over the affected lobe
(e)   ankle oedema.

R-6   The following is *not* a well-recognised complication of ulcerative colitis:

(a)   sclerosing cholangitis
(b)   carcinoma of the colon
(c)   enterocolic fistula
(d)   toxic megacolon
(e)   dehydration.

R-7   The following could shift the trachea to the right:

(a)   a large retrosternal goitre
(b)   a left pneumonectomy
(c)   a left lower lobe collapse
(d)   a left pneumothorax under tension
(e)   chronic right upper zone tuberculosis with fibrosis.

R-8   Patients with primary Sjögren's syndrome may develop:

(a)   gritty eyes
(b)   interstitial lung disease
(c)   a photosensitive skin rash
(d)   arthritis
(e)   parotid gland enlargement.

R-9   The following clinical situations would produce a normochromic normocytic anaemia:

(a)   renal failure
(b)   thalassaemia major
(c)   acute gastrointestinal haemorrhage
(d)   severe iron deficiency
(e)   active rheumatoid arthritis.

R-10   The following is/are feature(s) of hypertrophic cardiomyopathy:

(a)   asymmetrical septal hypertrophy
(b)   mitral regurgitation
(c)   sudden death
(d)   increased risk of infective endocarditis
(e)   systolic posterior motion of the mitral valve.

R-11 The following findings suggest that renal failure is chronic rather than acute:

    (a)   palpable kidneys
    (b)   hyperkalaemia
    (c)   a two-year history of nocturia
    (d)   signs of anaemia
    (e)   red cell casts in the urinary sediment.

R-12 A 19-year-old woman has mild mitral valve prolapse. The following is/are correct:

    (a)   she is likely to be asymptomatic
    (b)   a midsystolic click is always present
    (c)   a murmur is always present
    (d)   she should have an annual cardiac review
    (e)   signs of heart failure are likely to be present.

R-13 A 35-year-old healthy man who is a labourer presents with the acute onset of severe low back pain after lifting a heavy load. There are no neurological signs, but the patient is tender over L5. The most likely cause of his back pain is:

    (a)   spondylolisthesis
    (b)   septic discitis
    (c)   spinal canal stenosis
    (d)   ankylosing spondylitis
    (e)   herniation of a thoracic disc.

R-14 The diagnosis of Alzheimer's disease is most likely suggested by:

    (a)   poor memory for recent events
    (b)   a history of poorly controlled hypertension
    (c)   a stepwise deterioration in cognitive functioning
    (d)   difficulties with visuo-spatial tasks (copying, drawing)
    (e)   a marked change in personality with uncharacteristic aggressive outbursts.

R-15 The following nosocomial infections is/are transmitted by accidental parenteral exposure (e.g. needlestick injury):

    (a)   hepatitis C
    (b)   hepatitis A
    (c)   syphilis
    (d)   human immunodeficiency virus (HIV)
    (e)   cytomegalovirus.

R-16 Infection with HIV is associated with an increased risk of:

    (a)   peripheral neuropathy
    (b)   thrombocytopenia
    (c)   cancer of the lung
    (d)   dementia
    (e)   cerebral lymphoma.

R-17   A 79-year-old previously well man is brought to hospital with a three-day history of increasing confusion and urinary incontinence. Important factors contributing to his current illness may include:

(a)   pneumonia
(b)   constipation with faecal impaction
(c)   a urinary tract infection
(d)   a recent myocardial infarction
(e)   fever.

R-18   A 39-year-old woman presents with polyarthritis. Features which suggest that this is due to rheumatoid arthritis include:

(a)   symmetrical pattern of joint involvement
(b)   iritis
(c)   stiffness most marked in the evening
(d)   family history of ankylosing spondylitis
(e)   nodules over the extensor surfaces of her forearms.

R-19   The following is/are true of migraine:

(a)   the headache may be bilateral
(b)   it is more common in men
(c)   it is often associated with a positive family history
(d)   the headache is often associated with nausea
(e)   the headache may be preceded by homonymous hemianopia.

R-20   An 18-year-old man presents with acute arthritis in his right ankle. The following suggest a diagnosis of septic arthritis:

(a)   temperature of 40°C
(b)   history of a recent boil
(c)   recent new sexual contact
(d)   painless joint swelling
(e)   an injury to the ankle at football six hours previously.

R-21   The following symptoms or signs may be caused by an embolus within the left middle cerebral artery:

(a)   dressing apraxia in right-handed patients
(b)   right hemiparesis and deviation of the eyes to the left
(c)   motor dysphasia
(d)   loss of vision in the left eye
(e)   cortical blindness.

R-22   A 39-year-old male meat worker presents with an irregularly irregular pulse (due to atrial fibrillation) of two days' duration and an otherwise normal cardiovascular system examination. The following is correct:

(a)   he is likely to remain in atrial fibrillation
(b)   he is unlikely to have underlying structural heart disease
(c)   brucellosis should be excluded
(d)   ischaemic heart disease could *not* explain this problem
(e)   alcohol does *not* cause this problem.

R-23 Right heart failure may be associated with:

- (a) obesity
- (b) recurrent deep venous thrombosis
- (c) snoring loudly
- (d) an unrepaired atrial septal defect
- (e) chronic malaria.

R-24 The following phenomena occur in more than 50% of patients presenting with infective endocarditis:

- (a) retinal lesions
- (b) heart murmur
- (c) splenomegaly
- (d) splinter haemorrhages
- (e) haematuria.

R-25 Questions about risk factors are a routine part of history taking. The following activities put people at significant risk of developing disease:

- (a) smoking 15 cigarettes a day
- (b) drinking 15g of alcohol a day
- (c) eating butter
- (d) having a father who had a myocardial infarction at the age of 69 years
- (e) a single blood pressure reading of 170/75 mmHg immediately after exercise.

R-26 It is important to take a menstrual history because:

- (a) amenorrhoea is usually pathological
- (b) abdominal irradiation should be avoided in a woman who might be pregnant
- (c) pregnant women often need higher doses of therapeutic drugs because of pregnancy-induced induction of liver enzymes
- (d) ultrasound examinations are not safe in pregnancy
- (e) menstruation is affected by weight loss.

R-27 The following lung disorder(s) is/are related to asbestos exposure:

- (a) pleural plaques
- (b) predominant upper zone lung fibrosis
- (c) a pleural transudate
- (d) pneumothorax
- (e) widespread 0.5cm diameter nodular lung lesions.

R-28 The following occur(s) in Reiter's syndrome:

- (a) painless mouth ulcers
- (b) asymmetrical arthritis affecting the lower limbs
- (c) interstitial lung disease and fine inspiratory crackles
- (d) conjunctivitis
- (e) photosensitive skin eruption.

R-29   Primary generalised osteoarthritis is characterised by the following features:

  (a)   prolonged early morning joint stiffness
  (b)   bony swelling of the distal interphalangeal joints
  (c)   it more often affects women
  (d)   a positive family history
  (e)   bony swelling of the proximal interphalangeal joints.

R-30   Dementia in persons over 65 years of age:

  (a)   is associated with decreased life expectancy
  (b)   affects 75% of those over the age of 85 years
  (c)   is most frequently of sudden onset
  (d)   is usually due to Alzheimer's disease
  (e)   is generally reversible with treatment.

R-31   The syndrome of rash and arthritis or arthralgia is often associated with the following:

  (a)   hepatitis B
  (b)   serum sickness
  (c)   measles
  (d)   gout
  (e)   Ross River virus.

R-32   A 43-year-old Maori presents with the acute onset of arthritis in his right knee. He has had previous episodes of self-limiting arthritis in his lower limbs. Features which suggest that he suffers from gout include:

  (a)   his Maori origin
  (b)   a history of recent high alcohol intake
  (c)   presence of tophi
  (d)   self-limited nature of his arthritic attacks
  (e)   rigors.

R-33   A 19-year-old man develops a swollen right knee and Achilles tendonitis 12 days after an episode of diarrhoea due to *Shigella flexneri*. The following is/are correct:

  (a)   it will be possible to culture *Shigella flexneri* from the synovial fluid
  (b)   he may have urethritis
  (c)   the arthritis will resolve after about three months
  (d)   he is likely to be HLA-B27 positive
  (e)   he may have circinate balanitis.

R-34   A 22-year-old patient presents to hospital in coma following a motor bike accident. The following brainstem neurological sign(s) is/are important in assessing the patient's prognosis:

  (a)   the oculocephalic reflex (doll's eyes reflex)
  (b)   the palmomental reflex
  (c)   the jaw jerk
  (d)   the pupillary light reflex
  (e)   the corneal reflex.

R-35 Scabies:

    (a)   is caused by an insect
    (b)   nearly always affects the hands
    (c)   nearly always affects the head
    (d)   is very contagious
    (e)   infestation makes a sexual history relevant.

R-36 The following statements concerning peripheral neuropathy is/are correct:

    (a)   diabetes mellitus is the commonest cause in Western countries
    (b)   patients presenting with the clinical picture of mononeuritis multiplex may have an underlying vasculitis
    (c)   in demyelinating neuropathies weakness usually predominates over sensory loss
    (d)   marked slowing of motor conduction velocity and/or conduction block are characteristic findings in acquired demyelinating neuropathy
    (e)   it is well recognised that alcohol usually causes neuropathy even in well nourished individuals.

R-37 The following is/are typical clinical features of a left lateral medullary stroke:

    (a)   left limb ataxia
    (b)   right homonymous hemianopia
    (c)   left Horner's syndrome
    (d)   right trunk loss of pain and temperature
    (e)   aphasia.

R-38 A 56-year-old woman presents with headache, increasing shoe size, prognathism and the carpel tunnel syndrome. The following clinical features should be sought:

    (a)   hypertension
    (b)   bitemporal hemianopia
    (c)   glucose in the urine
    (d)   hypertrophy of ulnar nerves
    (e)   abdominal striae.

R-39 Psoriasis:

    (a)   is associated with arthropathy
    (b)   affects up to 2% of the population
    (c)   may result in intestinal malabsorption
    (d)   is an immune complex mediated disease
    (e)   is associated with pitting of the nails.

R-40 A man of 38 years presents with the sudden onset of a very severe headache and vomiting. He has neck stiffness. The following diagnosis is the *most likely*:

    (a)   trigeminal neuralgia
    (b)   temporal arteritis
    (c)   vertebral artery thrombosis
    (d)   migraine
    (e)   subarachnoid haemorrhage.

R-41   The following is/are typical clinical features in a 53-year-old patient presenting with idiopathic Parkinson's disease:

    (a)   incontinence of urine
    (b)   impairment of hand dexterity
    (c)   neck rigidity
    (d)   an unsteady gait
    (e)   muscle weakness.

R-42   Squamous cell carcinoma:

    (a)   sometimes metastasises
    (b)   may develop from a solar keratosis
    (c)   may develop in a chronic ulcer
    (d)   occurs frequently in renal transplant patients
    (e)   may be pigmented.

R-43   Malignant melanoma:

    (a)   rarely metastasises
    (b)   may develop from a mole
    (c)   may be familial
    (d)   is treated by wide excision
    (e)   may regress spontaneously.

R-44   Atopic eczema:

    (a)   may be associated with allergic rhinitis
    (b)   may be associated with allergic conjunctivitis
    (c)   may cause psoriasis
    (d)   is an autoimmune disease
    (e)   usually presents in adult life.

Figure R1

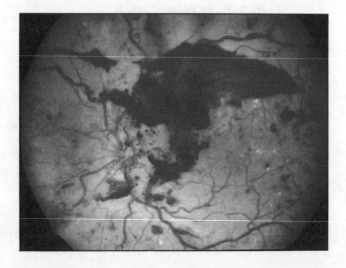

R-45   The retina in Photograph R.1 is from a diabetic patient. It is likely:

    (a)   that his vision is normal in this eye

    (b)   that better control of his blood sugar levels would have reduced the risk of development of these changes

    (c)   that he is likely to have been diabetic for only a short time

    (d)   that the new vessel formation will eventually help improve his vision

    (e)   any visual loss can be corrected with the appropriate spectacle lens.

R-46   The following conditions may often be diagnosed with some confidence from the characteristic facial appearance:

    (a)   diabetes insipidus

    (b)   acromegaly

    (c)   myxoedema

    (d)   Parkinson's disease

    (e)   mild-moderate mitral stenosis.

R-47   The following strongly suggest that a cardiac murmur is innocent:

    (a)   the patient has no cardiac symptoms

    (b)   the murmur is only audible to the consultant and there are no other signs

    (c)   the murmur is very short and diastolic

    (d)   a systolic thrill is palpable but only over a very small area of the praecordium

    (e)   the second heart is split but the splitting does not vary with respiration.

R-48   A fit looking 20-year-old basketball player presents with the sudden onset of sharp chest pain and dyspnoea. The examination may well reveal:

    (a)   reduced breath sounds over one of the upper zones of the chest

    (b)   a dull percussion note in the same area

    (c)   fine inspiratory crackles in the lung bases

    (d)   no signs at all since he is probably in the early period after a myocardial infarction

    (e)   a third heart sound.

R-49   The presence of bronchial breathing over the sternum:

    (a)   is always abnormal

         because

    (b)   bronchial breathing is diagnostic of lung consolidation.

R-50   If a patient presents with generalised pruritus the following conditions should be considered as possible causes:

    (a)   pregnancy

    (b)   cholestatic jaundice

    (c)   Addison's disease

    (d)   polycythaemia rubra vera

    (e)   acromegaly.

R-51   The characteristic skin colour changes of Raynaud's syndrome may be secondary to the following:

    (a)   working with jack-hammers
    (b)   scleroderma
    (c)   diabetes mellitus
    (d)   infective endocarditis
    (e)   vinyl chloride exposure.

Chapter 15

Answers

References are to *Clinical Examination, 3rd Edition.*

Chapter 1
The General Principles of History Taking

1-1 **Correct answers (a), (c), (d). Reference: Table 1.2.**
The great majority of cases of carcinoma of the lung occur in smokers. There is a dose-response relationship between the number of cigarettes smoked and lung cancer; compared with a non-smoker, the risk of lung cancer is increased up to 70-fold in two-packet a day smokers. Asbestos exposure is associated with squamous cell carcinoma or adenocarcinoma and the effect of smoking multiplies the risk. Peripheral vascular disease is rare in non-smokers. Coronary artery disease is much more common in smokers, but the risk in smokers is less in societies where the average serum cholesterol is lower. Chronic liver disease and diabetes mellitus are not associated with smoking, although the risk of vascular complications is much greater for diabetics who smoke.

1-2 **Correct answers (a), (c), (d). Reference: page 6 and Table 1.3.**
A standard measure of alcohol is 10g; this is the equivalent of one middy of beer or one nip of spirits. Forty grams a day, with two alcohol-free days a week, is considered the maximum safe level of alcohol consumption for men; 20g is considered the equivalent maximum safe level for women. Atrial fibrillation can be precipitated by consumption of large amounts of alcohol and is a common cause of atrial fibrillation in otherwise well young patients. In developed countries alcohol is the most common cause of chronic liver disease; hepatitis B or C (but not hepatitis A) can also cause chronic liver disease.

1-3 **Correct answer (c). Reference: page 299.**
The patient in this photograph looks thyrotoxic — this was confirmed on thyroid function testing. Patients with thyrotoxicosis commonly have diarrhoea and a preference for cold weather. Many have weight loss despite having a normal or better than normal appetite. Ankle oedema is not typical of thyrotoxicosis, but swelling of the ankles and legs can occur in hypothyroid patients. Severe chronic airflow limitation caused by smoking can be associated with slight lid retraction but not to the extent shown here.

1-4 **Both statements are true. Reference: page 4.**
Many drugs are teratogenic, particularly in the first and second trimesters of pregnancy — the time when pregnancy is least obvious to the casual observer. Radiological procedures should be avoided if at all possible in pregnant women because of the radiation risks to the fetus.

1-5 **Correct answers (a), (b), (c), (d). Reference: page 280.**
The photograph shows the typical facial rash of lupus erythematosus. A long history of rashes would support the diagnosis of lupus. The antihypertensive drug hydralazine can cause a lupus-like syndrome. Most patients with lupus have arthritis arthralgia, while 50% have renal tract symptoms (e.g. haematuria).

95

1-6   **Correct answers (b), (c), (d).**
This lesion is a tendon xanthoma. These lipid deposits are found in patients with familial hyperlipidaemia and are associated with premature coronary artery disease. Smoking further increases the patient's risk of coronary artery disease. Familial hyperlipidaemia may be associated with a family history of ischaemic heart disease.

1-7   **Correct answers (a), (c).**
Similar lesions can be found on extensor surfaces. On the eyelids they are called xanthelasma.

1-8   **Correct answer (d).**
It is unwise to ignore patients' claims about drug allergies, even if these seem 'far-fetched'. It is usually possible by questioning the patient to find out more about previous allergic reactions. The doctor needs to determine if they were likely to have been definite allergic reactions (e.g. urticaria, anaphylaxis), or merely side effects of a particular drug (e.g. nausea or diarrhoea are *not* allergic drug manifestations but common side effects).

Chapter 2
The General Principles of Physical Examination

2-1   **Correct answers (b), (e).**
By tradition, and for the benefit of right-handed examiners, patients are examined from the right side of the bed. The abdomen is best examined when the abdominal muscles are relaxed, which occurs when a patient lies flat. The cardiovascular system is best examined with the patient at 45 degrees, so that the height of the jugular venous pressure (JVP) can be estimated. Cranial nerves are best examined with the patient sitting up or sitting over the edge of the bed so that the head is roughly level with the examiner's head. Severe orthopnoea would prevent a patient being able to lie flat.

2-2   **Correct answer (e). Reference: page 14.**
Although a patient may look breathless and cardiac failure may be suspected, it is difficult to distinguish this from breathlessness due to respiratory disease just by inspection. All the other conditions should be recognised on inspection.

2-3   **Correct answer (b).**
Much information can be obtained by inspecting the hands before palpation is begun. However, the creaking sensation caused by the movement of inflamed or thickened tendons (tendon crepitus) must be felt to be appreciated.

2-4   **Correct answer (e). Reference: page 19.**
All of these can cause the skin to appear pale, but variations in skin pigmentation are very common and obviously not pathological unless due to vitiligo.

2-5   **Both statements are true. Reference: page 18.**
Cyanosis is caused by the presence of deoxygenated haemoglobin in superficial skin blood vessels; more than 50g/L of deoxygenated haemoglobin must be present to produce a bluish tinge. This cannot occur if the total haemoglobin level is low.

2-6   **Correct answers (a), (b), (d), (e). Reference: page 19.**
Peripheral cyanosis does not affect the tongue because this is a vascular area and is not usually exposed to low temperatures. Cyanosis of this type is due to the presence of

deoxygenated blood, present because of increased oxygen extraction by the tissues. Peripheral cyanosis occurs normally in peripheral parts of the body exposed to cold, and is a result of vasoconstriction, a heat conserving mechanism. Arterial occlusion, which eliminates or reduces blood supply to a region of the body, results in increased extraction of oxygen from the red blood cells remaining in the area. Central cyanosis implies reduction in oxygenation in the conduit arteries; peripheral cyanosis occurs because reduced amounts of oxygen are reaching the periphery rather than because of increased extraction in these circumstances.

2-7   **Correct answers (a), (b), (c), (d).**
Pallor may be a subtle sign of disease but is usually present in patients who are anaemic or have a reduced cardiac output. Pallor of the skin creases is considered to be a better sign of anaemia but cannot be relied on to make a diagnosis.

2-8   **Statement 1 is correct, statement 2 is false. Reference: page 18.**
In forms of congenital heart disease where unoxygenated blood is able to reach the systemic circulation, cyanosis will be present. This usually involves shunting of blood from the right side of the circulation to the left in the heart or in the lungs.

2-9   **Both statements are true. Reference: page 19.**
Some haemoglobin abnormalities result in differences in the colour of haemoglobin even when it is fully oxygenated.

2-10   **Correct answers (b), (c), (e). Reference: page 19.**
Medically defined shock includes reduction in cardiac output associated with hypotension. It can occur after large myocardial infarctions and as part of an anaphylactic response. It may also complicate Gram-negative sepsis.

2-11   **Correct answers (a), (b), (d). Reference: page 22.**
Cigarette smokers often have characteristic yellow discoloration of the fingers. The amount of discoloration depends more on the way cigarettes are held than on the number consumed. Infective endocarditis may produce a number of characteristic changes in the nails. Thyrotoxic patients may have separation of the nail from the nail bed — Plummer's nails.

Chapter 3
The Cardiovascular System

3-1   **Both statements are false. Reference: page 45.**
The height of the jugular venous pressure (JVP) can only be measured accurately with the patient at 45 degrees (or sitting upright if the JVP is very elevated).

3-2   **Correct answers (b), (c), (e).**
Not all patients with ischaemic heart disease have symptoms and some patients with severe coronary artery disease may not have angina even though abnormalities on the ECG may occur with exertion. The word 'angina' means 'choking' in Latin. Clinically, angina is a feeling of tightness in the chest predictably associated with exertion and relieved by rest. Angina is quite often *not* described as a pain. Although many patients have a history of pre-existing angina at the time of an infarct, infarction may be the first presentation of ischaemic heart disease. Some patients with angina have no chest pain but are aware of dyspnoea on exertion.

3-3   **Correct answers (b), (c), (e). Reference: page 26.**
Class IV symptoms are those that occur at rest. Sometimes angina is felt only as a discomfort in the throat. The recent onset of angina is considered an unstable period, as is the recurrence of angina at rest. Typically, angina is relieved fairly rapidly (within a few minutes) by sublingual nitrates, a useful clinical clue.

3-4   **Both statements are incorrect. Reference: page 25.**
Chest pain unrelated to exertion, even if described as a tightness, is considered atypical chest pain. Most cases of atypical chest pain are unrelated to coronary artery disease.

3-5   **Correct answers (b), (c), (d), (e). Reference: page 29.**
There are many causes of ankle oedema, but it is most often a local problem related to venous drainage in the leg. It tends to be worse later in the day because of the effect of gravity. The calcium channel antagonists (used to treat hypertension) are a common cause. Only rarely, particularly in isolation, is ankle oedema an early sign of heart failure. Ankle oedema may be a sign of deep venous thrombosis or hypoalbuminaemic states.

3-6   **Correct answers (b), (c), (d). Reference: page 28.**
There are numerous causes of cardiac failure of which ischaemic heart disease is only one. All of them can cause dyspnoea. The presence of orthopnoea in a dyspnoeic patient is suggestive of cardiac failure rather than respiratory disease. Dyspnoea following a myocardial infarction suggests the onset of cardiac failure and therefore of considerable myocardial damage. Many patients with valvular heart disease present with dyspnoea.

3-7   **Correct answers (b), (d), (e). Reference: page 29.**
Most palpitations caused by cardiac arrhythmias are of sudden onset and offset. Supraventricular tachycardia may be terminated by the Valsalva manoeuvre, but this is not effective for atrial fibrillation or ventricular tachycardia. Sinus tachycardia with a rate over 150 is unusual except during strenuous exercise. An awareness of the heart beating is not necessarily abnormal but can be alarming to patients.

3-8   **Correct answers (a), (c). Reference: page 30.**
Coronary artery disease is a common condition. A patient's risk is considered increased only if first degree relatives (that is, siblings or parents) have premature coronary artery disease. Smoking is an important risk factor.

3-9   **Correct answers (a), (b), (c), (d), (e). Reference: page 34.**
Clubbing may occur in any of these conditions. Even when gross it is not usually noticed by the patient. Clubbing takes at least 6 to 8 weeks to appear because subacute or chronic illnesses are responsible.

3-10   **Correct answers (c), (d). Reference: page 37.**
The new onset of atrial fibrillation usually causes symptoms, but may not always do so, particularly in elderly patients with conducting system disease in whom the ventricular rate is slow. In a patient with normal conduction, the ventricular rate is often more than 150 beats a minute. Because of differences in filling time related to varying R-R intervals, cardiac output varies from beat to beat and the pulse feels irregular in time and amplitude. There may be no evidence of other underlying heart disease particularly in young patients.

3-11   **Correct answers (b), (c), (d), (e). Reference: page 41.**
The width of the blood pressure cuff should be approximately two-thirds that of the upper arm. Not all upper arms are the same width. The first sound heard with the

stethoscope as the cuff is let down is called Korotkoff I and is by definition the systolic blood pressure. The diastolic blood pressure is said to have been reached when the Korotkoff sounds disappear — Korotkoff V. In patients with severe aortic regurgitation, Korotkoff IV (a muffled sound) is a more accurate indication of the diastolic blood pressure. The differences in the course of the arteries as they enter the arms can result in a variation in blood pressure of up to 10mmHg between arms in normal people.

3-12   Correct answers (a), (c). Reference: page 45.
The internal jugular vein usually runs a fairly straight course down to the right atrium. Movements of the atrium, the right sided valves and the right ventricle cause movements in the top of this column of blood. It is quite difficult to see the top of the column if the patient is lying flat. When a patient is in atrial fibrillation, atrial contraction is lost, which removes the *a* wave from the JVP. Blood flow through the right side of the heart and into the lungs increases during inspiration and the JVP usually falls with inspiration. The rise in JVP on inspiration is abnormal and is called Kussmaul's sign. Large *v* waves occur in patients with tricuspid regurgitation.

3-13   Correct answers (b), (e).
The apex beat is normally felt in the mid-clavicular line on the left side and if displaced is a reliable sign of cardiac enlargement in the absence of gross lung pathology. It is usually displaced in patients with significant cardiac failure. Patients with mitral stenosis may have a palpable first heart sound and their apex beat may feel tapping in quality. The first heart sound is usually soft in patients with mitral incompetence. The apex beat is not palpable in some people because of the shape of the chest wall.

3-14   Correct answer (e). Reference: page 48.
A thick chest wall or an over-inflated chest are the most common causes of an impalpable apex beat.

3-15   Both statements are true. Reference: page 52.
The causes of the heart sounds are controversial but the first heart sound (S1) appears to correspond to mitral and tricuspid valve closure.

3-16   Both statements are true. Reference: page 53.
The pulmonary component of the second heart sound (P2) is usually louder on inspiration because of increased venous return to the right atrium and right ventricle.

3-17   Correct answers (a), (b), (c), (d), (e). Reference: page 54.
A third heart sound (S3) represents an abnormality of cardiac filling. The combined effect of a first, second and third heart sound resembles the sound of a galloping horse. A third heart sound can be physiological in children and pregnant women. Otherwise, it is a reliable sign of heart failure.

3-18   Both statement are true. Reference: page 54.
A summation gallop sometimes heard in patients with tachycardia disappears if the heart is slowed by carotid pressure.

3-19   Correct answers (c), (d), (e). Reference: page 55.
Systolic heart murmurs may be physiological. In these cases they are probably due to turbulence in the main pulmonary artery or at the base of the great vessels. Mitral stenosis causes a diastolic murmur. Mitral regurgitant murmurs are typically pansystolic. The systolic murmur of mitral valve prolapse is usually middle and late systolic. Aortic stenosis produces an ejection systolic murmur.

3-20   Correct answer (a).
The bell of the stethoscope amplifies low pitched sounds such as the diastolic murmur of mitral stenosis.

3-21   Correct answer (d). Reference: page 36.
This is a photograph of tuboeruptive xanthomata over the elbow. They are typical of type III hyperlipidaemia.

3-22   Correct answer (a). Reference: Table 3.3.
Finger clubbing may be familial. It is not associated with coronary artery disease and is not diagnostic of any of the other conditions listed.

3-23   Correct answer (b). Reference: page 71.
Left atrial enlargement can be fairly reliably diagnosed on a chest X-ray and is characteristic but not diagnostic of mitral stenosis. The left ventricle is not enlarged until cardiac failure has supervened, which is a very late event. Not all stenosed mitral valves are heavily calcified on chest X-ray. Pulmonary plethora is more typical of left-to-right shunting. Widening of the mediastinum is usually related to disease of the ascending aorta.

3-24   Correct answer (d). Reference: page 93.
Patients with Marfan's syndrome are at risk of dilatation and dissection of the ascending aorta. This may be visible on a chest X-ray as widening of the mediastinum.

3-25   Correct answer (b). Reference: page 37.
The R-R interval in patients with atrial fibrillation always varies to some extent. Careful palpation of the pulse should reveal its irregularity even if the heart rate has been controlled with medication (e.g. digoxin). A patient with complete heart block will have a regular escape rhythm or an artificial pacemaker rhythm even if the atria are fibrillating.

3-26   Correct answers (a), (b), (c), (d), (e).
These fingers show splinter haemorrhages and vasculitic lesions which can occur in infective endocarditis. Dental work and invasive procedures are common causes of bacteraemia and may have been carried out up to three months before infective endocarditis is diagnosed. The presence of neurological symptoms suggests embolic events from the infected valve. Patients may have had rheumatic fever as children and hence have rheumatic heart disease.

3-27   Correct answers (a), (b), (c), (e).
Microscopic haematuria is common in a patient with infective endocarditis. Patients with prosthetic valves have a high risk of endocarditis. A major embolic event may abolish a peripheral pulse. A third heart sound suggests the occurrence of cardiac failure, a poor prognostic sign.

3-28   Correct answer (b). Reference: page 175.
Soft abdominal bruits are often heard near the splenic artery and are not considered significant. Abdominal aneurysms do not normally cause any noise. Vascular liver tumours may cause a bruit, but these are rare.

3-29   Both statements are false. Reference: page 57.
Venous hums commonly cause continuous murmurs near the base of the neck and are not pathological.

3-30   **First statement false, second statement true. Reference: page 79.**
An increase in peripheral resistance caused by squatting will reduce the gradient across the outflow tract in patients with hypertrophic cardiomyopathy (HCM) and decrease the intensity of a murmur.

3-31   **Correct answers (c), (d), (e). Reference: page 65.**
Although the cardiac output is not normal, blood pressure may be maintained until quite late in the course of this disease. Central cyanosis is also an unusual and late sign. Sinus tachycardia is commonly present and this may increase the cardiac output slightly. A loud third heart sound may be palpable over the apex and this is a reliable sign of cardiac failure. Mitral regurgitation is very common as the mitral valve ring dilates.

3-32   **Correct answers (a), (b), (e). Reference: page 66.**
Peripheral oedema is an important sign of right ventricular failure, but most patients with peripheral oedema do not have right ventricular failure. Tricuspid regurgitation occurs quite early in the course of the disease and large v waves may be visible in the neck. Tricuspid regurgitation is often not associated with any murmur. The liver tends to be enlarged and tender because of stretching of the liver capsule rather than hepatic infarction. Ascites may develop quite commonly.

3-33   **Correct answers (a), (b), (c), (e). Reference: page 66.**
Many patients presenting with myocardial infarction have no signs, but signs of cardiac failure indicate an adverse prognosis. Myocardial infarction may be complicated by a number of rhythm disturbances including atrial fibrillation, ventricular tachycardia and various levels of heart block. Chest pain may occur because of further angina or pericarditis as well as because of another infarct. Embolic stroke caused by embolisation of clot from the left ventricle is a not uncommon complication of myocardial infarction.

3-34   **Correct answer (b), (d), (e). Reference: page 67.**
Infective endocarditis may develop on a previously normal valve, particularly in drug addicts with right-sided endocarditis. Although Osler's nodes are characteristic of the condition, they are very rare. Splinter haemorrhages are more common. Prosthetic valve endocarditis is becoming an increasing problem.

3-35   **Correct answers (b), (c), (e). Reference: page 69.**
A great majority of patients with hypertension have no detectable underlying cause. Fourth heart sounds (S4) are common in moderately severe hypertension. Papilloedema is a sign of very severe hypertension requiring urgent treatment. Hypertension itself causes no symptoms. Cardiac failure is one of the complications of long-standing hypertension.

3-36   **Correct answers (a), (b), (d), (e). Reference: page 70.**
Obesity and alcohol consumption are associated with hypertension; renal artery stenosis and Cushing's syndrome are important but relatively rare causes of hypertension. Most commonly, no cause for hypertension can be detected (essential hypertension).

3-37   **Correct answers (b), (c), (e). Reference: page 71.**
Severe mitral stenosis is present if the valve area is less than $1cm^2$. Rheumatic fever remains the most common cause of mitral stenosis. The first heart sound (S1) is loud because the mitral valve cusps remain open late, and shut forcefully when ventricular systole occurs. Characteristically these patients have a late diastolic murmur with presystolic accentuation. There is a considerable risk of the development of atrial fibrillation in patients with mitral stenosis or mitral regurgitation.

3-38   Correct answers (a), (e). Reference: page 73.
Mitral valve prolapse is very common. It is often but not always associated with a mid-systolic click; there may be a click and no murmur. It very uncommonly progresses to cause significant mitral regurgitation and to affect life expectancy.

3-39   Correct answers (b), (e). Reference: page 74.
Exertional syncope is characteristic of aortic stenosis, but only late in the disease. Rheumatic fever can cause aortic stenosis, but is by no means the only cause. Associated aortic regurgitation is quite common, particularly if looked for with sensitive Doppler ultrasound equipment. Cardiac failure is a late sign in aortic stenosis.

3-40   Correct answers (c), (d), (e). Reference: page 76.
A congenitally abnormal aortic valve is a rare cause of aortic regurgitation. Aortic regurgitation is tolerated for long periods before it causes symptoms. Typically the pulse is collapsing because of the wide pulse pressure.

3-41   Correct answer (c). Reference: page 73.
Mitral valve prolapse is now the most common cause of pure mitral regurgitation.

3-42   Correct answer (b). Reference: page 48.
Valve replacement surgery produces a median sternotomy scar. Closed mitral valvotomy can be performed through a lateral thoracotomy incision. Heterograft or human valves do not make mechanical valve sounds. Only patients with mechanical prostheses require anticoagulation with warfarin following valve replacement.

3-43   Correct answer (a). Reference: page 87.
Cardiomegaly as seen on chest X-ray may be due to left ventricular hypertrophy, cardiac enlargement or a pericardial effusion.

3-44   Correct answer (a). Reference: page 80.
Dilated cardiomyopathy usually results in left ventricular failure, and the most common presentation is with dyspnoea. There is often an element of biventricular failure and some patients present with hepatic congestion and peripheral oedema.

3-45   Correct answer (d). Reference: page 69.
Hypertension itself does not produce symptoms even though some patients feel they can tell when their blood pressure is elevated. Mild hypertension can often be controlled by reducing salt and alcohol intake, losing weight and regular exercise. A single high blood pressure recording, particularly if it is only a little elevated, may well not be significant. At least three abnormal readings need to be taken on separate days before a diagnosis can be made. In the majority of cases, there is no specific underlying identifiable cause for hypertension. Many patients can have their blood pressure controlled with a single drug, but some need a combination of different classes of antihypertensive medications.

3-46   Correct answers (b), (c), (d), (e). Reference: page 36.
Tendon xanthomata are common in patients with hyperlipidaemia, particularly types IIa, III and V. Although these patients have a high risk of coronary artery disease and typically have relatives with coronary artery disease, they usually do not have established coronary artery disease at the time of the occurrence of the lesions. The lesions tend to be present over extensor surfaces. Hypothyroidism can be associated with hyperlipidaemia and occasionally with xanthomata.

3-47   Correct answers (b), (c), (e). Reference: page 78.
Pulmonary stenosis is usually congenital but occasionally may not present until adult life. The murmur is usually harsh and loud and is associated with a thrill in the pulmonary area. The murmur tends to increase on inspiration as blood flow through the lungs

increases. Signs of right ventricular hypertension may be present including a fourth heart sound (S4).

3-48   Correct answers (a), (d), (e). Reference: page 80.
Dilated cardiomyopathy often presents with no obvious cause, but many of these cases may be due to a viral myocarditis. Heavy alcohol consumption and certain inherited conditions such as dystrophia myotonica can be the cause.

3-49   Both statements are correct. Reference: page 81.
Dissection of the ascending aorta may involve the origins of one of the coronary arteries and lead to its occlusion. These patients may present with myocardial infarction.

3-50   Correct answers (c), (d), (e). Reference: page 81.
Ventricular septal defect (VSD) is not an uncommon congenital abnormality, but is less common than bicuspid aortic valve (which is said to occur in 2% of the population). These patients rarely present with central cyanosis, since shunting of blood in the heart is from left to right. The murmur tends to be harsh and associated with a systolic thrill at the left sternal edge. A myocardial infarct involving the septum may sometimes lead to a VSD; these patients develop a new murmur usually some days after the onset of the infarct. A small VSD may never involve enough shunting to cause cardiac symptoms.

3-51   Correct answers (b), (d), (e). Reference: page 82.
The characteristic sign of an atrial septal defect (ASD) is fixed splitting of the second heart sound. The second heart sound normally varies with inspiration, since the pulmonary component of the second heart sound (P2) is delayed as right ventricular output increases because of increased venous return. In patients with an ASD, P2 is delayed throughout the respiratory cycle and in most cases the second heart sound is widely split but there is no respiratory variation. Increased flow through the pulmonary valve causes a systolic ejection murmur. Mitral regurgitation is associated with mitral valve abnormalities that occur with ostium primum defects. Occasionally patients do not present until later in life when heart failure has often supervened.

3-52   Both statements are true. Reference: page 82.
When the ductus arteriosus fails to close shortly after birth, continuous shunting occurs from the descending aorta to the pulmonary artery unless pulmonary artery pressure has risen to above systemic pressure; this is usually a late development.

3-53   First statement true, second statement false. Reference: page 84.
Shunting at any level between the pulmonary and systemic circulations can eventually lead to pulmonary hypertension. If pulmonary pressures rise above systemic, shunting reverses so that right-to-left shunting occurs. Unoxygenated blood is then able to reach the systemic circulation.

3-54   Correct answers (b), (e). Reference: page 85.
The right heart border on chest X-ray is usually formed by the inferior and superior vena cavae and right atrium. The right ventricular border is not usually visible on the posterior-anterior (PA) chest X-ray. The curve of the aortic arch is usually visible above the left hilum and is called the aortic knuckle. An abnormal cardiothoracic ratio is one exceeding 50%, although this is not a very accurate way of measuring heart size. Severe valvular heart disease may be associated with valvular calcification, particularly if the valvular disease is rheumatic. The absence of calcium, however, does not exclude a significant lesion. The left and right main pulmonary arteries form the hilar shadows on chest X-ray.

3-55   Correct answers (a), (b), (c), (d). Reference: page 89.
Cardiac enlargement on chest X-ray may be due to left ventricular hypertrophy, where increased left ventricular muscle mass makes the heart appear large. It is difficult

to distinguish this from left ventricular dilatation. It may be possible on the lateral chest X-ray to distinguish right ventricular from left ventricular dilatation, but both make the heart look large on a PA film. Pericardial effusion may cause globular enlargement of the cardiac shadow. The heart size usually looks normal in patients with dextrocardia; the apex points to the right (unless the radiographer has just mislabelled the X-ray).

Chapter 4
The Respiratory System and Breast Examination

4-1   **Correct answers (a), (b), (c), (d). Reference: page 97.**
Some patients with asthma may have only a dry cough without symptoms of wheeze or dyspnoea. Bronchiectasis is associated with a productive cough of often voluminous amounts of unpleasant sputum present since childhood. The angiotensin-converting enzyme inhibitors, as a class of drugs, may cause chronic cough in up to 10% of patients who take them. Patients with cardiac failure sometimes present with a dry cough or a cough productive of clear sputum. Cystic fibrosis in adults is associated with a productive cough that has been present since childhood.

4-2   **Correct answers (a), (b), (c), (e). Reference: page 98.**
Haemoptysis can be an alarming symptom and may turn smokers into ex-smokers. Particularly in children, the forgotten inhalation of a foreign body can be a cause of haemoptysis. Carcinoma of the lung is the most feared cause in adults, but it can also occur in patients with pneumonia, or pulmonary infarction following a pulmonary embolus.

4-3   **Correct answers (a), (b), (c), (e). Reference: page 99.**
The classification of dyspnoea is similar to the classification of angina. Patients with class IV symptoms are breathless even at rest. Some patients with asthma may be dyspnoeic even when no wheeze is audible in the chest. Patients with chronic airflow limitation in particular may just have reduced breath sounds on auscultation. Paroxysmal nocturnal dyspnoea is a more typical symptom of cardiac failure than of asthma. Dyspnoea can be the result of anxiety or lack of physical fitness; it is not always due to a cardiac or respiratory abnormality. Pulmonary embolism should always be considered a possible cause in a patient who presents with dyspnoea, particularly if it is of sudden onset and occurs a few days after a surgical operation.

4-4   **Correct answers (a), (c), (d), (e). Reference: page 102.**
Contact with avian antigens and pathogens may cause respiratory disease (e.g. psittacosis) even when the birds are as far away as a nextdoor neighbour's garden. Exposure to dust (e.g. asbestos) at any stage in a patient's life is significant. Some eye drops for glaucoma contain beta-blockers which may be systemically absorbed and result in bronchospasm in patients with chronic airflow limitation or asthma. The total number of cigarettes smoked may be relevant even if the patient has stopped smoking. This is particularly true if cessation of smoking has been recent. Some cytotoxic drugs (e.g. bleomycin) may cause pulmonary fibrosis.

4-5   **First statement true, second statement false.**
Finger clubbing may be associated with hypertrophic pulmonary osteoarthropathy in a proportion of cases but is by no means always present.

4-6   **First statement true, second statement false. Reference: page 105.**
Staining of the fingers of cigarette smokers is not considered a reliable sign of the number of cigarettes smoked, because it depends a lot on the way the cigarette is held. The cause of this staining is tar, not nicotine, which is colourless.

4-7   **Both statements are true. Reference: page 108.**
Patients treated for tuberculosis before modern antimicrobial drugs were available may
have had a thoracoplasty with removal of a number of ribs from one side of the chest
and collapse of the affected lung. This causes severe chest deformity. It is not performed
any more and indeed is not useful in treating tuberculosis.

4-8   **Correct answers (a), (c), (d), (e). Reference: page 108.**
The crackling sensation caused by air in the subcutaneous tissues is diagnostic of
subcutaneous emphysema. It does not occur in normal people. The most common cause
is pneumothorax where air from a ruptured lung is able to track into the chest wall, but
it can also occur following thoracotomy or rupture of the oesophagus.

4-9   **Correct answers (a), (d), (e). Reference: page 108.**
Watching movement of the clavicles from behind is the best way of assessing upper lobe
expansion. Lower lobe expansion is best judged from behind. Reduced wall movement
may be due to a pneumothorax, collapse, consolidation or pleural effusion.

4-10   **Correct answers (a), (b), (c), (d), (e). Reference: page 110.**
Percussion note over normal lung is defined as resonant and indeed has a resonant
quality. Percussion over fluid causes a very dull note, and percussion over large air-filled
spaces (e.g. a pneumothorax or bowel) is more resonant than over normal lung. The
percussion note over an area of lung consolidation is dull, but not as dull as the note
over a fluid-filled area. The percussion note over the liver is dull and the upper border
of the liver may be defined in this way.

4-11   **Correct answers (a), (b), (d), (e). Reference: page 111.**
Sounds heard over normal lung are defined as vesicular. The sound is said to be similar
to that of the wind rustling through leaves. The inspiratory phase is normally longer
than the expiratory one and there is not normally a gap between inspiration and
expiration. Breath sounds heard over the main bronchi are described as bronchial. They
have a more hollow sound than vesicular breath sounds. This sound is conducted
through solid lung and is thus heard over consolidated lung tissue. An even more hollow
sound may be heard over a cavity. This is described as amphoric.

4-12   **Both statements are true. Reference: page 113.**
It is more accurate to describe breath sounds as normal or reduced than to talk about air
entry. The breath sounds do not correlate directly with the amount of air entering and
leaving the lungs.

4-13   **Correct answers (b), (c), (e). Reference: page 113.**
Breath sounds are reduced or absent over a pleural effusion and are reduced in patients
with overexpanded lungs and emphysema. There are usually no breath sounds over a
significant sized pneumothorax and breath sounds over the main bronchi are bronchial.

4-14   **Both statements are false. Reference: page 113.**
Wheezes tend to be louder on expiration since forced expiration tends to cause narrow-
ing of the airways and therefore more obstruction to airflow.

4-15   **Correct answers (a), (d). Reference: page 114.**
The airways obstruction caused by asthma limits airflow particularly in expiration.
Airflow limitation may be associated with wheeze but in many cases, particularly when
the condition is chronic, there are simply reduced breath sounds. In patients with severe
asthma, breath sounds may be soft and wheezes almost inaudible because of reduced air
flow; the wheezes may get louder as the patient improves. Obstruction of a single
bronchus, often caused by carcinoma of the lung, can produce an expiratory wheeze

which is unaffected by coughing and has a single note. This is described as monophonic. Patients with airflow limitation may present with cough rather than dyspnoea or may be asymptomatic.

4-16   Correct answers (a), (b), (d). Reference: page 114.
High-pitched interrupted sounds are usually described as crackles (or crepitations); lower pitched crackles have traditionally been called rales. Mid-inspiratory crackles are more typical of airflow limitation. Fine inspiratory crackles associated with pulmonary fibrosis have been compared with the sound of Velcro strapping. Coarse crackles are typical of chronic lung infection like bronchiectasis and are not a normal finding.

4-17   Correct answers (a), (b), (d), (e). Reference: page 114.
Friction rubs are caused by the rubbing together of inflamed serosal surfaces. Pericarditis is a common cause. Pulmonary infarction results in an area of localised pleural inflammation and can cause a rub. Clinically these patients have pain on deep inspiration as the serosal surfaces rub against each other; the roughened surfaces may rarely cause a palpable grating sensation.

4-18   Correct answer (a), (d). Reference: page 115.
Vocal resonance is a way of testing the lung's ability to transmit sound. Consolidated lung transmits high frequency sounds better than normal lung. This tends to make speech more clearly audible. Although consolidated lung lying above a pleural effusion may cause increased vocal resonance, sounds are generally reduced when auscultation is performed over the effusion itself. Whispering pectoriloquy is detected by asking the patient to whisper "sixty six"; it is a sign of greatly increased vocal resonance. Auscultation over normal lung while the patient speaks is associated with attenuation of high frequencies.

4-19   Correct answers (b), (c). Reference: page 115.
Pulmonary hypertension is rarely caused by acute respiratory diseases, but may occur in patients with chronic pulmonary thromboembolism. It may also occur in pulmonary fibrosis. Although they can be chronic, lung abscesses do not affect enough of the pulmonary vascular bed to lead to pulmonary hypertension.

4-20   Both statements are false. Reference: page 116.
The normal forced expiratory time is three seconds or less. Patients with chronic airflow limitation have a prolonged forced expiratory time.

4-21   Correct answers (a), (b), (d), (e). Reference: page 116.
A peak flow meter measures the maximum velocity of exhaled air. Patients should be taught to puff into the device. A normal man would be expected to have a PEFR of 600 litres a minute. Patients with asthma have a reduced PEFR because of airflow limitation. Normal values depend on a patient's age, gender and height.

4-22   Correct answers (a), (b), (d). Reference: page 116.
The basic measurements made with a spirometer include the volume of air that can be expired from the lung from maximum inspiration to maximum expiration. The forced expiratory volume expired in one second (FEV_1) is usually measured. The forced vital capacity (FVC) is the volume that can be expired after maximum inspiration. Usually the highest reading of these measurements is taken as the most accurate. In normal young men approximately 80% of the total forced vital capacity can be expelled in one second. The FEV_1/FVC ratio tends to fall with age.

4-23   Correct answers (a), (c). Reference: page 118.
The percussion note over an area of consolidation is dull, but not stony dull. A stony dull note is more characteristic of pleural effusion. Bronchial breath sounds are nor-

mally heard over an area of consolidation due to conduction of airways noise from the main bronchi; there is improved conduction of high-pitched sounds and vocal resonance increases. Lung expansion is reduced on the affected side since the consolidated lung is not filled with air. Amphoric breath sounds are heard over a cavity.

4-24   Correct answers (a), (b), (d). Reference: page 120.
A small collection of fluid in the pleural space or pleural effusion may have no noticeable affect on lung capacity and cause no symptoms. Bleeding into the pleural space is called a haemothorax, and leakage of chyle or lymphatic fluid is called a chylothorax. Pus in the pleural space is called empyema. Fluid in the pleural space may compress overlying lung, so that bronchial breathing is detectable. Pleural effusions do not always imply lung disease. They may occur for many reasons including cardiac failure and disseminated malignancy.

4-25   Both statements are true.
A spontaneous or traumatic pneumothorax enables air to leak into the chest wall and make its way into the subcutaneous tissues.

4-26   Correct answers (b), (d). Reference: page 121.
The lung on the side of the chest involved with a pneumothorax does not expand normally. Chest wall expansion is also reduced because normal lung is not present in this area. Breath sounds are absent or reduced. The percussion note tends to be hyper-resonant. Small pneumothoraces do not interfere with lung function sufficiently to cause cyanosis. A tension pneumothorax where air continues to leak from the lung under pressure may interfere with lung function and cardiac output, resulting in hypotension; this is a medical emergency.

4-27   Correct answers (a), (b), (d), (e). Reference: page 121.
Patients with bronchiectasis usually have a very productive cough that has persisted since childhood. Finger clubbing may occur in advanced disease, but is not always present. There is often associated bronchospasm and evidence of airways obstruction. Cystic fibrosis is sometimes the underlying abnormality since this condition involves abnormal clearance of mucus.

4-28   Correct answers (b), (c), (e). Reference: page 122.
Most asthmatics have a hyperinflated chest, but inability to speak because of dyspnoea suggests a severe attack and cyanosis is a very late sign. Breath sounds are reduced in patients with severe asthma. A reduction in blood pressure of more than 20mmHg on inspiration (pulsus paradoxus) is a sign of severe disease and should be taken very seriously.

4-29   Correct answers (b), (c), (d). Reference: page 122.
Traditionally patients with chronic airflow limitation are divided into those with predominant emphysema ('pink puffers') and those with predominant chronic bronchitis and large airway obstruction ('blue bloaters', because of cyanosis and oedema). This distinction may not always be entirely appropriate, but emphysematous patients are less often cyanosed than those with chronic bronchitis. They tend to expire through partly closed lips because this increases the expiratory pressure and tends to keep airways open. Smoking is the most common cause of both conditions and overinflation of the chest occurs in both. The accessory muscles of respiration may be in obvious use.

4-30   Both statements are true. Reference: page 123.
Reduced gas transfer and hypoxia are common in patients with significant pulmonary fibrosis. The cause is not the thickening of the alveolar membrane but mismatching of perfusion and ventilation within the lungs.

4-31   Correct answers (b), (d). Reference: page 123.
Pulmonary fibrosis is not associated with cigarette smoking but is quite often caused by mineral dust inhalation. The condition is chronic and, unlike chronic airflow limitation, may be associated with finger clubbing. Typically, fine inspiratory crackles are heard at the lung bases. Rheumatoid arthritis is associated with pulmonary fibrosis involving particularly the lower lobes.

4-32   Correct answers (b), (c), (d). Reference: page 124.
Tuberculosis has recently become more common in developed countries, partly due to immigration and human immunodeficiency virus (HIV) infection. Early in the course of the disease, patients may have no abnormal signs in the chest. Typical symptoms include fevers and night sweats. The symptoms are usually chronic. Tuberculosis may present with typical changes of erythema nodosum on the legs. Close contacts of patients with tuberculosis are at increased risk of infection and must be examined and investigated.

4-33   Correct answers (a), (c), (d). Reference: page 124.
Structures in the mediastinum can be compressed by primary carcinoma of the lung or involved mediastinal lymph nodes. Mediastinal compression is not a feature of emphysema or chest injuries, but a chest injury leading to a pneumothorax may cause mediastinal shift. Dermoid cysts are typically midline structures and may compress the mediastinum, as may a large retrosternal goitre.

4-34   Correct answers (a), (b), (d). Reference: page 125.
Superior vena caval (SVC) obstruction and associated increases in venous pressure in the head may cause exophthalmos. Causes of SVC obstruction, including lymphoma and carcinoma of the lung, may result in supraclavicular lymphadenopathy. Stridor is common as a result of compression of the trachea rather than laryngeal nerve involvement. Interruption of the sympathetic innervation may result in a Horner's syndrome. The jugular venous pressure is elevated because of problems with venous return from the head.

4-35   First statement true, second statement false. Reference: page 125.
Hyponatraemia may occur in patients with carcinoma of the lung. This usually occurs with small (oat) cell carcinoma, not squamous cell carcinoma, and is the result of inappropriate antidiuretic hormone release.

4-36   Correct answers (c), (d). Reference: page 126.
The non-caseating granulomas typical of sarcoid do not contain mycobacteria. Granulomas may occur anywhere in the body. Patients may go on to develop pulmonary fibrosis. Lupus pernio is a well-known association. Splenomegaly does not usually occur.

4-37   Correct answers (a), (b), (c), (d), (e). Reference: page 126.
Massive pulmonary embolism may suddenly obliterate such a large proportion of the pulmonary arterial circulation that cardiac arrest occurs. On the other hand, very small pulmonary emboli may cause no symptoms. Immobilised patients are at risk of pulmonary embolism because of venous pooling in the pelvis and legs. Recurrent or acute pulmonary embolism may be the cause of dyspnoea and haemoptysis. Recurrent pulmonary embolism can be the cause of right ventricular failure.

4-38   Correct answers (b), (d), (e). Reference: page 133.
Although nipple retraction occurs typically in carcinoma of the breast there are numerous other causes. Infiltration of the skin with tethering of sweat glands causes the typical *peau d'orange* appearance in advanced disease. Paget's disease of the nipple is due to

malignant infiltration of the nipple. It is most important to establish whether there is involvement of draining lymph nodes. Green discharge from the nipple is typical of mammary duct ectasia.

4-39 **Correct answers (c), (d). Reference: page 106.**
The trachea is sensitive, and forceful compression of it is very uncomfortable. The normal trachea lies almost exactly in the midline. Collapse of one of the upper lobes typically causes deviation of the trachea to that side. The tracheal tug is a downward movement of the trachea on inspiration in patients with overinflated lungs. It can be felt by placing the finger gently on the surface of the trachea. Assessment of the tracheal position is not helped by getting the patient to swallow a glass of water.

4-40 **Correct answers (b), (e). Reference: page 110.**
Percussion directly over the clavicle produces a percussion note from the upper lobe on that side. Percussion in this area normally produces a resonant note. There are no underlying cardiac structures to cause dullness. A pleural effusion causes lower chest dullness but rarely dullness over the upper lobes. A pneumothorax, if large, causes a hyper-resonant note particularly over the upper lobes.

4-41 **Correct answers (a), (d). Reference: page 109.**
Lower lobe expansion is assessed by placing the hands as shown in this photograph except that the thumbs should not contact the chest wall. This reduces their movement and makes the assessment less accurate. The side with reduced movement is usually the one with pathology. Pulmonary fibrosis tends to cause an overall reduction in expansion. Chronic airflow limitation is associated with reduced expansion in all areas.

4-42 **Correct answers (b), (d). Reference: page 109.**
The examiner has his hand over the base of the heart well away from the apex beat. A palpable pulmonary component of the second heart sound (P2) may be felt in this area and suggests pulmonary hypertension. The thrill of a ventricular septal defect may be felt in this area but is only felt in systole. Pulmonary stenosis produces a systolic thrill palpable over the base of the heart. Subcutaneous emphysema can often be felt in this area when it is present.

4-43 **Correct answers (b), (d), (e).**
These photographs show correct examination of the chest. The thumbs should be lifted off the chest wall. The thumbs should normally move apart at least 5cm as the patient breathes in deeply. Reduced chest wall movement is likely to be found if the patient has chronic airflow limitation. Consolidation will reduce expansion on the affected side.

4-44 **Correct answers (a), (b).**
Chest expansion is best assessed from behind the patient by looking for movement of the clavicles. Upper lobe fibrosis will reduce clavicular movement on both sides. Supraclavicular lymphadenopathy will not be visible unless the nodes are grossly enlarged. The movement of the clavicles usually appears symmetrical.

4-45 **Correct answer (d). Reference: page 126.**
Sarcoidosis can affect many parts of the body but the lungs are most commonly involved. Clinical cardiac involvement occurs fairly rarely.

4-46 **Correct answer (d). Reference: page 123.**
Despite assertions by smokers who may feel that their chronic bronchitis is really related to exposure to industrial dusts or gases, smoking is the most common cause.

4-47   Correct answer (a). Reference: page 97.
Asthma may occasionally present, especially in children, with just a dry cough. Cough may sometimes be due to anxiety rather than lung pathology. Bronchiectasis by definition causes a productive cough. Heart failure may sometimes present as a cough, particularly a nocturnal cough when a patient lies down. Some drugs such as the angiotensin-converting enzyme inhibitors can be associated with a dry cough, but cough is not a feature of antibiotic sensitivity.

4-48   Correct answer (b).
Metabolic acidosis causes deep and rapid respirations as the body compensates to increase blood pH by removing carbon dioxide.

4-49   Correct answer (c). Reference: page 108.
Patients who have had radiotherapy usually have small tattoo marks at the corners of the irradiated area. The skin often appears erythematous and thickened. Increased skin pigmentation may be present.

4-50   Correct answer (c). Reference: page 86.
Dextrocardia is a very uncommon condition. It is more frequent for the markings on the chest X-ray film to be incorrect than for a patient to have dextrocardia. The other conditions listed do not reverse the position of the apex.

4-51   Correct answer (c). Reference: page 87.
The left main bronchus, although visible on the chest X-ray, does not form part of the cardiac border.

Chapter 5
The Gastrointestinal System

5-1   Correct answer (b). Reference: page 140.
The patient described has typical symptoms of peptic ulcer disease, but burning epigastric pain can also be a symptom of gastro-oesophageal reflux disease. The irritable bowel syndrome characteristically causes crampy mid or lower abdominal pain that is relieved by defaecation or is associated with disturbances of defaecation. Oesophageal adenocarcinoma would be very unusual in a young patient and would not be expected to cause burning epigastric pain. Carcinoma of the transverse colon may very rarely cause upper abdominal pain but again the character of the pain in this case would be atypical. Biliary pain from gallstones is typically severe constant pain that lasts for hours and occurs in episodes; gallstones do not cause vague dyspepsia.

5-2   Correct answer (a). Reference: page 141.
An increased appetite in combination with weight loss is much less common than anorexia with weight loss. However, hypermetabolic states can cause the combination of weight loss and increased appetite (e.g. thyrotoxicosis). Depression, occult malignancy (e.g. pancreatic or lung cancer) and anorexia nervosa usually cause weight loss with loss of appetite (anorexia). Tumour necrosis factor and other cytokines contribute to the weight loss associated with malignancy. Diseases causing steatorrhoea (e.g. coeliac disease, chronic pancreatitis or cystic fibrosis) can be associated with weight loss occurring despite an increased food intake.

5-3   Correct answers (b), (c), (d), (e). Reference: page 142.
Odynophagia is a condition that can occur when there is any severe inflammation of the oesophagus. Therefore, oesophageal ulceration, ingestion of caustic substances, viral oesophagitis and fungal oesophagitis can all cause odynophagia.

5-4   **Correct answers (a), (b), (d), (e). Reference: page 143.**
Malabsorption of fat causes fatty stools (steatorrhoea) which are pale coloured, extremely smelly, tend to float in the toilet bowl and are very difficult to flush away. Not only fat but also fat-soluble vitamins will be malabsorbed in this situation. This can lead to manifestations of vitamin deficiency such as easy bruising (from vitamin K deficiency), night blindness (vitamin A deficiency), bone pain (vitamin D deficiency) and peripheral neuropathy (vitamin E deficiency). Examination of the mouth may reveal glossitis and angular stomatitis (related to water-soluble vitamin deficiencies — malabsorption of B_2, B_6, B_{12}, thiamine or niacin), intraoral purpura (from vitamin K deficiency) or hyperkeratotic white patches (from vitamin A deficiency).

5-5   **Correct answer (d). Reference: page 146.**
In this case, the patient has melaena stools suggesting upper gastrointestinal tract bleeding, from the oesophagus, stomach or duodenum. Less often right-sided colonic bleeding and rarely small bowel bleeding cause melaena. The physical sign of pallor suggests anaemia which can be secondary to blood loss. Non-steroidal anti-inflammatory drugs (NSAIDs) may cause ulceration in the gastrointestinal tract; therefore, peptic ulcer is the correct answer.

5-6   **Correct answers (a), (b), (c), (d). Reference: page 148.**
As the skin and gastrointestinal tract have a common origin from the embryoblast, a number of diseases can present with both skin and gut manifestations. In the Peutz-Jeghers syndrome, pigmented macules on the hands, feet and lips are apparent and haematomatous polyps in the stomach, small bowel and colon occur; very rarely adenocarcinomas may occur in this syndrome. In porphyria cutanea tarda, vesicles occur on the sun-exposed skin including the hands. This is due to deficiency of uroporphyrin decarboxylase. Many of these patients have hepatitis C infection; some have chemically induced liver disease (e.g. by hexachlorobenzene). Excess alcohol consumption may also contribute to the disease. In the carcinoid syndrome, a tumour secretes excess serotonin leading to flushing, telangiectasia of the skin and watery diarrhoea. Hepatomegaly is frequently present because of metastatic carcinoid tumour; the abnormal liver is no longer able to break down serotonin sufficiently to prevent the clinical manifestations occurring. In dermatitis herpetiformis, pruritic vesicles occur on the knees, elbows and buttocks. This condition is associated very strongly with coeliac disease. Patients with acanthosis nigricans have brown or black skin papillomas, usually in the axillae. This condition is not associated with gastro-oesophageal reflux but can occur with bowel cancer, acromegaly or diabetes mellitus.

5-7   **Correct answer (a). Reference: page 153.**
White nails (leuconychia) are found in hypoalbuminaemic states such as occur in chronic liver disease. Fever, bowel cancer, porphyria cutanea tarda and thyrotoxicosis do not cause hypoalbuminaemia and therefore do not cause leuconychia.

5-8   **Correct answers (a), (b), (d), (e). Reference: page 187.**
There are many signs of chronic liver disease which need to be kept in mind when the gastrointestinal system examination is being performed. These signs include: palmar erythema (reddening of the palms of the hands affecting the thenar and hypothenar eminences); jaundice manifesting as scleral icterus; spider naevi, which consist of central arterioles from which radiate numerous small vessels that look like spiders' legs; bruising resulting from inadequate clotting factor production; scratch marks due to severe itch with jaundice; leuconychia; clubbing; and hepatic flap (asterixis) that occurs in hepatic failure. Dupuytren's contracture, however, is a sign of alcoholism but not necessarily of liver disease; Dupuytren's contracture can also occur in manual workers and can be familial.

5-9   Correct answer (b). Reference: page 167.
There are a number of causes of enlargement of the liver that need to be remembered. Massive hepatomegaly below the umbilicus can occur as a result of metastatic liver disease; the lumps of tumour may be felt on the surface of the liver. Massive fatty infiltration can occur with alcoholic liver disease. Myeloproliferative disease and right heart failure are other causes. Alcoholic cirrhosis in the absence of fatty infiltration usually leads to a shrunken liver. Gallstones do not cause hepatomegaly unless there is biliary obstruction. A caput Medusae refers to prominent veins on the abdominal wall that flow away from the umbilicus in patients with intrahepatic portal hypertension. This is a very rare sign and usually only one or two veins can be seen.

5-10   Correct answers (a), (c), (d), (e). Reference: page 169.
Enlargement of the liver and spleen is an important finding. Haematological disease such as lymphoma or leukaemia can be a cause. Viral infections, including infectious mononucleosis, cytomegalovirus and acute viral hepatitis may also cause hepatosplenomegaly. Portal hypertension due to chronic liver disease is an important cause. However, colonic cancer metastatic to the liver does *not* lead to enlargement of the spleen in the absence of portal hypertension.

5-11   Correct answer (c). Reference: page 171.
There are many possible causes of a mass in the left iliac fossa. One needs to consider all the possible anatomical structures below the palpating finger that could produce a mass. As the mass was not tender, an abscess is unlikely. The absence of pulsation suggests it is not a vessel. The most important physical sign in this case is that the mass indents on being pressed firmly, suggesting that this is in fact stool. A colonic cancer or polyp would not be expected to indent. However, it would still be very important in this case to perform a colonic examination (e.g. colonoscopy) to exclude a colonic malignancy.

5-12   Correct answer (d). Reference: page 173.
Shifting dullness is an important sign to try to elicit, if dullness in the flanks is detected on percussion of the abdomen. To elicit the sign, percuss out to the left flank until you detect dullness on percussion. The patient should then be asked to roll towards you on the right and percussion is repeated after a minute or so to determine if the dull area has become resonant, suggesting a fluid shift.

5-13   Correct answers (a), (b), (c), (d), (e). Reference: page 160.
Causes of abdominal distension can be thought of in relation to the 5 'Fs': faeces, fluid, fetus, flatus and filthy big tumour (or phantom pregnancy). The irritable bowel syndrome can cause visible abdominal distension although the mechanism is unclear. Very severe constipation may lead to partial or complete large bowel obstruction and therefore distension. A pelvic tumour may grow large enough to cause an abdominal mass.

5-14   Correct answer (e). Reference: page 174.
Bowel sounds need to listened for during the routine physical examination. A complete absence of bowel sounds over a three minute period occurs with paralytic ileus.

5-15   Correct answer (d). Reference: page 178.
Rectal examination should always be performed as part of the gastrointestinal system examination unless there is a very good reason to defer it. Not only may rectal pathology be diagnosed, but the prostate gland can also be examined for evidence of nodules (e.g. prostatic cancer) or enlargement (e.g. prostatic hyperplasia). The cervix is felt on the anterior wall of the rectum, not the posterior wall. Rectal examination may be of value in any patient with lower gastrointestinal tract symptoms including diarrhoea which may be due, for example, to a villous adenoma in the rectum.

5-16   Correct answers (a), (b). Reference: page 184.
The urinary and stool changes that occur in jaundice need to be understood. An increase in conjugated bilirubin in the urine and absence of urinary urobilinogen suggest total biliary obstruction (cholestasis). Cholestasis may occur in cases of acute or chronic liver disease. A raised urobilinogen can occur with acute liver damage where the liver is unable to re-excrete the urobilinogen absorbed from the bowel. A raised urobilinogen may also occur with increased red cell breakdown as occurs in haemolytic jaundice.

5-17   Correct answer (b). Reference: page 142.
Dysphagia means difficulty in swallowing and can occur for solids or liquids or both. Dysphagia for solids is a feature of gastro-oesophageal reflux associated with stricture formation. External obstruction of the oesophagus from a large goitre can produce dysphagia. Stress is not a proven cause of dysphagia. Dysphagia may occur together with painful swallowing (odynophagia), as with ulceration of the oesophagus.

5-18   Correct answer (a). Reference: page 188.
An hepatic flap (asterixis) is an important sign of liver failure and should always be looked for in patients with suspected liver disease. It is characterised by a jerky, irregular flexion-extension movement of the wrist and metacarpophalangeal joints; it is *not* a fine regular tremor. Asterixis does not occur with barbiturate overdose alone. Hepatic encephalopathy does not cause jaundice, but underlying liver disease can cause both jaundice and a flap. Hepatic encephalopathy does not cause Dupuytren's contractures, but these may occur with alcoholism.

5-19   Correct answer (d). Reference: page 190.
Causes of fat malabsorption (steatorrhoea) include diseases that affect the mucosal lining of the small bowel (e.g. coeliac disease, Crohn's disease). Diseases that may interfere with normal mixing in the small bowel (e.g. after gastrectomy) or diseases that affect the delivery of lipase (e.g. chronic pancreatitis) or bile salts to the small bowel can also cause fat malabsorption. Ulcerative proctitis could not cause steatorrhoea.

5-20   Correct answers (a), (b), (c), (d). Reference: page 191.
Systemic signs of inflammatory bowel disease are important and include erythema nodosum, clubbing, iritis and a non-deforming arthritis. Cardiac failure is not a feature of inflammatory bowel disease.

5-21   Correct answers (a), (d), (e). Reference: page 151.
Photograph 5.1 (a and b) show multiple telangiectasia involving the lips and tongue. Multiple telangiectasia occur in the syndrome hereditary haemorrhagic telangiectasia (or Rendu-Osler-Weber syndrome). Telangiectasia can be found anywhere on the skin including the nail beds. This is an autosomal dominant condition and although relatively rare it is a cause of bleeding from the gastrointestinal tract. The Peutz-Jeghers syndrome refers to freckle-like spots on the buccal mucosa and fingers and toes that are associated with hamartomas of the small bowel and colon. Telangiectasia are not a sign of underlying chronic liver disease.

5-22   Correct answers (a), (b), (c).
Photograph 5.2 shows generalised abdominal distension with eversion of the umbilicus; the typical findings in massive ascites. If ascites is suspected this should be confirmed by percussion. Other causes of abdominal distension such as fat or retained faeces would not be expected to cause eversion of the umbilicus. Causes of ascites include cirrhosis of the liver with portal hypertension, malignant disease, infection (e.g. tuberculosis), pancreatitis and the Budd-Chiari syndrome (hepatic vein thrombosis). Neither cholecystitis nor diverticulitis cause this clinical picture.

5-23   Correct answers (a), (b), (c), (d), (e). Reference: page 176.
The differential diagnosis of a groin mass includes both femoral and inguinal hernias. A swelling that lies medial to and above the pubic tubercle is likely to be a direct inguinal hernia. This is typically a soft lump that can be pushed back into the abdominal cavity and conducts a palpable impulse when the patient coughs. A femoral hernia occurs lateral to and below the pubic tubercle, 2cm medial to the femoral pulse, and does not involve the inguinal canal. It is usually small and firm and so can be mistaken for a lymph node. An undescended testis or a lipoma can also cause a groin mass.

5-24   Correct answer (a). Reference: page 187.
The man described in this case has ascites, because there is shifting dullness on abdominal examination. However, he also has signs of chronic liver disease with clubbing, leuconychia, multiple spider naevi and palmar erythema, which strongly suggests that the most likely underlying diagnosis is cirrhosis of the liver. The nephrotic syndrome can cause ascites but not signs of chronic liver disease. Malignant disease involving the liver and peritoneal cavity, and myxoedema and pancreatitis may cause ascites but not signs of chronic liver disease.

5-25   Correct answer (b).
Positioning the patient for a gastrointestinal system examination is important. Lying the patient comfortably flat with one pillow allows optimal examination of the abdomen. Hepatic encephalopathy is due to decompensation of liver function in cases of chronic or acute liver failure. To test for an hepatic flap (asterixis), ask the patient to sit up and then stretch out his or her arms in front, separating the fingers and extending the wrists. Look for jerky, irregular flexion-extension movements at the wrist and metacarpophalangeal joints. A similar flap can occur with cardiac, respiratory or renal failure or hypoglycaemia. The rectal examination and examination with the sigmoidoscope are usually done with the patient in the left lateral position (or less often the knee-chest position). To examine for an inguinal hernia, it is best to ask the patient to stand up. In a male, indirect inguinal hernias can be sought by invaginating the scrotum. If the spleen is initially not palpable, it is best to ask the patient to roll over towards you (on the right side) and repeat the palpation to determine if there is mild splenomegaly.

5-26   Correct answers (b), (e). Reference: page 182.
One should never miss an opportunity to examine the patient's stools or vomitus if this material is available. Melaena refers to black tarry appearing stools that have a particularly offensive and distinct smell that distinguishes them from normal stool. Melaena occurs when blood is digested either by acid or colonic bacteria, and therefore melaena can occur from upper or lower gastrointestinal tract bleeding. However, bleeding from lesions in the lower left colon will not cause melaena. Steatorrhoea from fat malabsorption can cause very pale, offensive, smelly and bulky stools that are difficult to flush away. Coffee ground vomitus refers to the appearance of old blood clot in the vomitus, although similar appearances can occur with iron tablets or red wine. Haematochezia means the passage of bright red blood per rectum; while this most commonly occurs with disease of the anorectum or left colon it can occur with rapid bleeding from more proximal sites. Other causes of black stools include bismuth, licorice, iron tablets and charcoal, but these substances do not cause a tarry appearance or an offensive smell.

5-27   Correct answers (a), (b), (c), (d), (e). Reference: page 165.
The liver may be normal but palpable because it is pushed down by the overinflated lungs of a patient with emphysema. A subdiaphragmatic collection such as a subphrenic abscess can also cause ptosis of the liver. Riedel's lobe is a tongue-like projection of liver from the inferior surface of the right lobe. It can be quite large. Hydatid disease due to echinococciasis can rarely cause a palpable mass in the liver. Chronic constrictive

pericarditis can cause hepatomegaly due to increased venous pressure transmitted via the hepatic vein. Right ventricular failure can cause tender hepatomegaly due to increased venous pressure (the liver may be pulsatile if there is also tricuspid regurgitation).

5-28   Correct answer (e). Reference: page 181.
Testing the stools for blood is part of the physical examination and is useful when evaluating patients with suspected anaemia, gastrointestinal bleeding or colorectal cancer. With the guaiac test, stool is placed on guaiac-impregnated paper; in the presence of blood, phenolytic oxidation occurs causing a blue colour. A positive test is not diagnostic of colorectal cancer and can occur because of bleeding from other lesions. False positive guaiac test results can occur from haem in red meat and from peroxidase or catalase present in various foods, as well as from iron supplements. Currently, testing the stool for blood in asymptomatic people may be of value in screening for colonic cancer in older adults, but is not recommended in people under 40 years of age.

5-29   Correct answers (a), (b), (c), (d), (e). Reference: page 159.
Creamy white patches in the mouth suggest *Candida albicans* (thrush). HIV infection may lead to thrush because of immunosuppression. Diabetes mellitus can also predispose to thrush, therefore the urine should be tested for sugar. Thrush can affect the nail beds of the fingers or toes. Thrush may also spread to the oesophagus producing dysphagia and odynophagia. Alcoholism can cause immunosuppression and hence thrush may be found in these patients; other signs of alcoholism may include fetor, Dupuytren's contractures, a coarse tremor, peripheral neuropathy and memory loss.

5-30   Correct answers (a), (b). Reference: page 170.
If a mass is found in the left hypochondrium, it is important to decide if it is a spleen or a kidney. The mass identified in this question is likely to be the kidney, as there was a space between the mass and the left costal margin (which would not be expected with the spleen) and the mass moved inferiorly on inspiration (the spleen usually moves inferomedially on inspiration). Unlike the spleen, the kidney is ballottable. The kidney often has a resonant percussion note over it because it lies posterior to loops of gas-filled bowel, unlike the spleen. While a friction rub may occasionally be heard over the spleen, this is not heard over the kidney because it is too posterior. Gastric carcinoma is very rarely palpable and would usually produce a fixed mass in the epigastrium. A pancreatic pseudocyst has to be extremely large to be palpable, would not move on inspiration and is usually felt as a rounded swelling above the umbilicus.

5-31   Correct answer (c). Reference: page 168.
The presence of ascites is always abnormal. The edge of the normal liver can often be felt by the skilled examiner just below the right costal margin, when the patient breathes in deeply. The spleen, however, must be enlarged to be palpable. The absence of bowel sounds suggests the presence of paralytic ileus. A succussion splash is often audible for a few hours after a meal in normal people.

5-32   Correct answer (c). Reference: page 170.
Physical signs are unusual when patients have peptic ulceration unless a complication (such as bleeding or perforation) has occurred. Sometimes there is epigastric tenderness but this is not of diagnostic value. *Helicobacter pylori* does not cause a rash.

5-33   Correct answers (a), (c), (d). Reference: page 158.
The characteristic smells of exhaled ketones and of uraemia are difficult to describe but easy to remember. The unpleasant stale smell of cigarette smoke should remove any idea of glamour associated with this addiction. Oesophageal reflux can cause an acid

taste in the mouth, but the smell of the breath is not helpful. Pernicious anaemia does not affect the breath.

5-34   Correct answers (d), (e). Reference: page 189.
Hypotension occurs when compensating mechanisms such as vasoconstriction are unable to maintain blood pressure in the face of blood loss. In most patients this is likely to occur well before half the blood volume has been lost. Bright red rectal bleeding may occasionally occur as a result of upper gastrointestinal haemorrhage if the rate of bleeding has been very high. The decision to transfuse a patient depends on haemodynamic abnormalities and the measured haemoglobin level rather than the presence of melaena. A patient with melaena will, however, require admission to hospital for observation and upper gastrointestinal endoscopy. NSAIDs are a common cause of gastrointestinal bleeding. Anaemia caused by gastrointestinal blood loss may precipitate angina in patients with pre-existing coronary artery disease.

5-35   Correct answers (a), (c). Reference: page 156.
Vitamin deficiency can be caused by malabsorption. This may result in clotting abnormalities and purpura (vitamin K deficiency). Leucoplakia is a whitish thickening of the mucosa which can be due to poor dental hygiene; it is premalignant. Crohn's and coeliac disease can cause malabsorption and can result in aphthous ulceration. True macroglossia occurs with acromegaly, amyloid disease, tumours or Down's syndrome.

5-36   Correct answers (a), (b). Reference: page 160.
Cimetidine (but not the other H_2-receptor antagonists) and spironolactone (a diuretic often used in cirrhotics) are associated with gynaecomastia. Gynaecomastia can occur occasionally in patients with chronic hepatitis or cirrhosis (often alcoholic) because of failure of the liver to remove oestrogens.

5-37   Correct answers (a), (b). Reference: page 168.
Carcinoma of the head of the pancreas causes early obstruction to bile flow and therefore jaundice which may be accompanied by an enlarged gallbladder. Primary carcinoma of the gall bladder is a rare cause of enlargement. Primary liver disease is not associated with gall bladder enlargement. Gallstones (cholelithiasis) causes fibrosis of the wall of the gallbladder so that enlargement is unusual (Courvoisier's law).

5-38   Correct answers (a), (b). Reference: page 191.
Erythema nodosum and pyoderma gangrenosum (an ulcerating lesion often found on the trunk) are among the classical skin changes found in some patients with inflammatory bowel disease (usually ulcerative colitis or colonic Crohn's disease).

5-39   Correct answers (a), (c), (d). Reference: page 191.
Toxic megacolon or toxic dilatation of the colon is a feared complication of severe inflammatory bowel disease. Typically there is abdominal pain with high fever, tachycardia and dehydration. Abdominal tenderness, distension, and signs of peritonism are the important signs to look for.

5-40   Both statements are false. Reference: page 179.
The prostate gland is normally palpable in men of all ages. It is a firm, but not hard, bilobed mass. It gradually enlarges with advancing age. Carcinoma of the prostate is very common in men in their eighth and ninth decades. Irritative (e.g. dysuria) or obstructive (e.g. difficulty in voiding) symptoms or haematuria are common presenting symptoms. Characteristically there is a hard, irregular palpable nodule. It begins most often in the lateral lobes but benign disease may also arise here. Lymphoedema of the legs or scrotum (from pelvic lymph node involvement) or signs of spinal cord compression from metastatic disease can occur with advanced disease.

Chapter 6
The Genitourinary System

6-1   **Both statements are true. Reference: page 201.**
Although red discoloration of the urine suggests haematuria, there are other causes including the consumption of beetroot.

6-2   **Correct answers (a), (b), (c), (e). Reference: page 201.**
Prostatic enlargement due to hyperplasia is probably the commonest cause of urinary obstruction in men and occurs increasingly frequently as they get older. Obstructive symptoms include a decreased urinary stream, difficulty in starting micturition, post-void dribbling and a sense of incomplete emptying of the bladder. Urinary incontinence may develop because of obstruction and overflow. Note that irritative symptoms (dysuria, frequency and urgency) can be caused by infectious or malignant conditions as well as by prostatic enlargement Ureteric calculi can cause obstruction which is usually very painful. Nocturia is also a common symptom because of incomplete evacuation of the bladder.

6-3   **Correct answers (b), (c), (d). Reference: page 203.**
Although chronic renal failure can present with oliguria, some patients pass large volumes of urine. Nocturia is common because of an inability to concentrate the urine. Chronic renal failure often causes vomiting, pruritus and a bleeding diathesis. Hypotension is not a common presenting feature.

6-4   **First statement true, second statement false. Reference: page 203.**
Cardiogenic shock is a cause of acute renal failure because of reduced perfusion of the kidneys. Creatine kinase can cause renal damage, but not in the amounts released from the damaged myocardium.

6-5   **First statement true, second statement false. Reference: page 207.**
The typical sallow complexion of uraemic patients is probably due to a combination of the accumulation of the urinary pigments in the skin combined with anaemia.

6-6   **Correct answers (a), (c), (d). Reference: page 207.**
When chronic renal disease results in proteinuria and thus hypoalbuminaemia, nail beds opacify leaving a rim of pink nail at the top. Clubbing is not associated with chronic renal failure. Half-and-half nails involve a distal brown or red arc, and occur in renal failure or cirrhosis. Mee's lines are single white bands across the nail and occur in renal failure, arsenic poisoning or with other severe illnesses. Onycholysis (separation of the nail from its bed) does not occur in renal disease but occurs in thyrotoxicosis or psoriasis.

6-7   **Correct answers (a), (c), (d). Reference: page 208.**
Coagulation and platelet abnormalities make bruising common in patients with renal failure. Uraemic frost is the deposition of a fine white powder on the skin; this is very rare, but may occur in terminal chronic renal failure. Pruritus leading to scratch marks may be due to calcium or phosphate deposition or both. Urinary pigments (or urochromes) can cause skin pigmentation. Areas of depigmentation are not associated with renal disease.

6-8   **Correct answers (c), (d), (e). Reference: page 209.**
A normal right kidney may be palpable in very thin patients; transplanted kidneys are usually palpable since they are placed more anteriorly. Nephrectomy scars may be missed on examination of the abdomen unless the back is inspected. It can sometimes

be difficult to distinguish an enlarged spleen from a palpable left kidney. If both kidneys are enlarged, one should suspect polycystic kidney disease or hydronephrosis. Other causes of bilateral renal enlargement are uncommon.

6-9   Correct answer (b). Reference: page 169.
Ballotting of the kidney involves brisk flexing of the fingers of the hand placed posteriorly so that the kidney floats anteriorly. A normal right kidney may sometimes be felt this way. The liver is not ballottable (unless there is gross ascites) and renal transplants are placed too superficially to be ballotted.

6-10   Correct answers (a), (b). Reference: page 203.
When trauma leads to significant injury of the limbs, abdomen or thorax, bleeding can occur externally or into the tissues themselves and lead to hypovolaemia. Muscle injury releases myoglobin into the blood. This is a renal toxin and can cause acute renal failure. Hypertension is unlikely after severe injury and is not likely to cause renal failure acutely. Pelvic fracture itself is not a cause of renal failure unless the injuries have caused hypovolaemia. Small pulmonary emboli can cause hypotension acutely, but not usually renal failure.

6-11   Correct answer (b). Reference: page 209.
Peritoneal dialysis fluid is not rapidly absorbed but is drained in and out of the peritoneal cavity. Very large polycystic kidneys may make the abdomen appear distended. Ascites may occur in the nephrotic syndrome but is not a feature of renal failure *per se*. Renal transplants are usually unilateral. Although ascites is common in patients with hepatic failure, it is not diagnostic of this condition.

6-12   Correct answers (a), (c), (d). Reference: page 211.
Renal tenderness can be elicited by gently striking the renal angle with the fist. This is called Murphy's kidney punch. Glomerulonephritis may lead to the nephrotic syndrome with gross proteinuria, resulting in hypoalbuminaemia and oedema. Patients with osteomalacia may have widespread bony tenderness. Nephrectomy scars are surprisingly posterior and may not be seen when the patient lies on his or her back. The kidneys are not palpable posteriorly.

6-13   Correct answer (d). Reference: page 211.
Secondary carcinoma is a very rare cause of renal failure. An enlarged bladder can be felt by palpating the abdomen. Constipation is common and hard faeces are not a useful sign of renal impairment. Prostatic hyperplasia is a common cause of urinary obstruction in elderly men and an enlarged prostate can be felt on rectal examination. The ureters are not palpable.

6-14   Correct answers (c), (d). Reference: page 211.
Renal failure does not lead to peripheral oedema unless hypoalbuminaemia is present or there is salt and water retention. Characteristically patients with hyperuricaemia due to renal failure do not have gout. Gout, however, can be a cause of renal failure. Peripheral neuropathy may complicate long-standing renal failure. Pruritus may occur in chronic renal failure because of secondary hyperparathyroidism.

6-15   Correct answers (a), (b), (d). Reference: page 210.
Polycystic kidney disease in adults (autosomal dominant) usually causes hypertension (75%) and the presence of hypertension indicates a worse prognosis. Subarachnoid haemorrhage due to a berry aneurysm is also an association. A ruptured berry aneurysm typically causes severe headache and often sudden loss of consciousness. Some of these patients may have hepatic or rarely splenic cysts. Carotid bruits and proximal myopathy are not recognised associations with polycystic disease.

6-16   **Correct answers (a), (c), (d). Reference: page 212.**
Normal urine has a smell suggestive of ammonia. The ingestion of asparagus may make the urine smell like asparagus. Antibiotics can also be smelt in the urine.

6-17   **Correct answers (a), (c), (e). Reference: page 212.**
Very dilute urine may appear colourless. This can be due to drinking large amounts of fluids or to inadequate secretion of anti-diuretic hormone in diabetes insipidus. There are numerous causes of red discoloration including ingestion of beetroot. Intravascular haemolysis of red cells in huge numbers can lead to the presence of haemoglobin in the urine. This occurs in severe falciparum malaria, where it is called blackwater fever. Infection of the urinary tract may make the urine appear cloudy.

6-18   **Correct answer (d). Reference: page 213.**
Dipstick testing of the urine may detect amounts of protein less than 150mg. This is + proteinuria and is not always abnormal. Bence-Jones protein is not detected by chemical dipsticks. There is not normally any sugar detectable in the urine. The presence of ketones in a diabetic patient raises the possibility of ketoacidosis. These sticks, however, react only to one of the ketones: acetoacetic acid.

6-19   **Correct answer (e). Reference: page 213.**
Patients with the nephrotic syndrome lose large amounts of protein in their urine and characteristically develop hypoalbuminaemia, oedema and hyperlipidaemia. More than 3.5g of protein is present in the urine daily. The condition is not usually associated with large kidneys.

6-20   **Both statements are true. Reference: page 215.**
Early morning urine is concentrated, and the urinary sediment in concentrated urine is more likely to contain casts than dilute urine.

6-21   **Correct answer (d). Reference: page 218.**
When a scrotal mass appears to be part of the testis, a tumour is the most likely cause. Syphilitic gummas are very rare and cysts of the epididymis are translucent.

6-22   **Correct answer (e). Reference: page 219.**
There are many causes of bloody vaginal discharge, but menstruation is, of course, the most common.

6-23   **Correct answers (c), (d). Reference: page 219.**
The cervix normally points towards the posterior vaginal wall. The ovaries are not usually palpable unless enlarged. The uterus can normally be well defined by palpation. Pregnancy causes a smooth enlargement of the uterus and this must always be considered in a patient of child-bearing age. The normal uterus is not tender.

Chapter 7
The Haematological System

7-1   **Correct answers (a), (b), (c). Reference: page 223.**
Iron deficiency anaemia is usually due to blood loss, most often from the gastrointestinal tract. For example, this is how colonic cancer may first manifest. The presence of symptoms of peptic ulceration suggests the possibility of a bleeding peptic ulcer. Rectal bleeding and melaena should be asked about; melaena suggests significant upper gastrointestinal tract bleeding. An early menopause is likely to be associated with

less menstrual bleeding and therefore less iron loss. Repeated blood donations, at least in Western countries, would be an unusual cause of anaemia since the haemoglobin is checked before each donation.

7-2   Correct answer (c). Reference: page 224.
Weakness, lethargy, exertional dyspnoea and fatigue are all common symptoms of anaemia because of reduced oxygen supplies to the tissues. Easy bruising is not a sign of anaemia itself, but may be caused by thrombocytopenia, platelet dysfunction (e.g. aspirin), coagulation disorders (e.g. liver disease or haemophilia), or loss of skin elasticity (senile ecchymoses).

7-3   Correct answers (a), (b), (c), (d), (e). Reference: pages 223, 238.
There are many possible causes of anaemia. A comprehensive history may give important clues. Aspirin may be associated with peptic ulceration and hence blood loss with iron deficiency. Malignancy can be associated with the anaemia of chronic disease. Rheumatoid arthritis may cause anaemia by a number of mechanisms including chronic disease, blood loss (from use of non-steroidal anti-inflammatory drugs) and Felty's syndrome. Previous gastric surgery may result in failure to produce intrinsic factor and reduced absorption of vitamin B_{12}. A recent change in bowel habit may be the first symptom of colonic cancer which can cause occult bleeding from the gastrointestinal tract.

7-4   Correct answer (d).
Pernicious anaemia is an autoimmune disease characterised by failure to absorb vitamin B_{12} because of lack of intrinsic factor (due to destruction of parietal cells by a chronic gastritis) rather than a failure to ingest vitamin B_{12}. Only very strict vegans are at any risk of failure to ingest sufficient vitamin B_{12}. Pernicious anaemia is associated with macrocytosis on the blood film, whereas iron deficiency is associated with microcytosis. Vitamin B_{12} tablets are not used for pernicious anaemia since vitamin B_{12} is not well absorbed in patients who lack intrinsic factor. Before vitamin B_{12} was available in its pure form, patients were encouraged to eat huge amounts of liver, which has a high concentration of vitamin B_{12} but this is not currently recommended. Pernicious anaemia is an uncommon cause of anaemia compared with iron deficiency.

7-5   Correct answers (a), (b), (c), (e).
The general inspection of a patient with suspected haematological disease may reveal clues to the diagnosis. The racial origin is relevant as haematological diseases such as thalassaemia are more common in southern Europeans and South East Asians. The presence of jaundice may suggest that significant haemolysis has been occurring. Scratch marks may be associated with pruritus which can occur with some forms of lymphoma and myeloproliferative disease. Polyarthritis, particularly if it is in a rheumatoid pattern, may be associated with anaemia, as mentioned above. Obesity itself is not associated with haematological disease.

7-6   Correct answer (d).
Patients with iron deficiency anaemia may occasionally present with koilonychia but this is not the only cause of the condition; fungal infections of the nails can occasionally be the explanation. Anaemic patients may have pallor of the nail beds, but this is also dependent on skin pigmentation and is not diagnostic. Pallor in the palmar creases is a more helpful sign, but again may be present in normal people. Anaemic patients with rheumatoid arthritis may have Felty's syndrome. In this case, rheumatoid arthritis is associated with splenomegaly and neutropenia. Gouty tophi may be an indication of increased urate production from a myeloproliferative or lymphoproliferative disease.

7-7   Correct answers (a), (b), (d), (e).
Petechial haemorrhages are usually related to thrombocytopenia or platelet dysfunction. Immune thrombocytopenic purpura (ITP) characteristically presents with this sign. Chronic renal failure may also cause platelet dysfunction and can be associated with petechial haemorrhages. Paracetamol does not affect platelet function, unlike aspirin. Hypersplenism can result in sequestration of platelets in the spleen and, therefore, thrombocytopenia. Meningococcal septicaemia is another important cause of petechial haemorrhages. In this case they are due to damage to small blood vessels.

7-8   Correct answer (c).
Elderly patients have fragile skin and subcutaneous tissue as a result of a loss of skin elasticity. They are at risk of damage to small blood vessels from fairly minor skin trauma. This is called senile purpura.

7-9   Correct answers (b), (d), (e).
Christmas disease (haemophilia B) is a clotting condition due to Factor IX deficiency. It was first identified in a family whose surname was 'Christmas'. Von Willebrand's disease is the most common inherited bleeding disorder and is due to decreased or dysfunctional von Willebrand factor, a glycoprotein. It causes less severe bleeding problems than Factor VIII deficiency (haemophilia A). Haemophilia A patients tend to present with haemorrhage into joints rather than with subcutaneous bruising.

7-10   Correct answers (b), (c), (d).
The epitrochlear lymph nodes are *not* usually palpable. The most common cause of enlargement is infection of the hand or arms. Para-aortic lymph nodes are rarely palpable even in thin patients when they are enlarged. Inability to feel them certainly does not indicate that they are of normal size. It is unusual for normal lymph nodes to be more than 1cm in diameter. Malignant disease is not the most common cause of lymph node enlargement; local infection is a more common cause.

7-11   Correct answers (b), (c), (e).
Inguinal nodes may become chronically enlarged because of recurrent infections of the legs, but they are not usually very hard or very large. Lymphoma causes firm or rubbery enlargement of lymph nodes, often in more than one area. Normal lymph nodes are mobile; fixation to underlying structures suggests malignant infiltration. Lymph nodes enlarged secondary to infection may often cause inflammation of overlying skin. A routine part of the examination of the breasts is assessment of the draining lymph nodes. Abnormal lymph nodes in the axilla in a patient with carcinoma of the breast suggests that spread has occurred.

7-12   Both (a) and (b) are true.
Conjunctival pallor is a more reliable sign of anaemia than pallor elsewhere in the body.

7-13   Correct answers (c), (d), (e).
Gum hypertrophy can occur in some malignancies, particularly monocytic leukaemia, but it is not a feature of anaemia. Patients with severe vitamin C deficiency (scurvy) often have swollen bleeding gums and their teeth may fall out. Badly fitting false teeth are a common cause of gum ulceration. Infections in the mouth and gums are common in patients with immune deficiency (e.g. the acquired immune deficiency syndrome (AIDS)).

7-14   Correct answers (a), (b), (d), (e).
Bony tenderness suggests that a patient may have bone marrow infiltration or a secondary malignant deposit in the bone. Traditionally, the spine is tapped with the edge of the fist. Obviously the blows must not be struck hard enough to cause pain. Squeezing the

sternum with the heel of the hand is another approach. Multiple myeloma is not the only cause of marrow infiltration and bony tenderness; others include leukaemia, lymphoma and metastatic malignancy.

7-15   Correct answers (a), (b), (c), (e).
Lymphadenopathy of more than one or two groups of nodes may occur in patients with lymphoma, acute viral infections such as infectious mononucleosis, sarcoidosis and systemic lupus erythematosus. Digoxin is not associated with lymphadenopathy.

7-16   Correct answers (a), (b), (c).
Leg ulcers may occur in haematological diseases associated with abnormal viscosity. Patients with thalassaemia, polycythaemia and sickle cell anaemia are all at risk of developing this problem. They may also occur when viscosity increases in certain conditions such as cold exposure in patients with cryoglobulinaemia. Leg ulcers are not a feature of iron deficiency or macrocytosis.

7-17   Correct answers (a), (c), (d).
Vitamin B_{12} deficiency is associated with a number of neurological and haematological manifestations (e.g. subacute combined degeneration of the cord, peripheral neuropathy, optic atrophy, dementia and macrocytic anaemia). These do *not* include proximal myopathy or hepatic problems.

7-18   Correct answers (a), (b), (d).
Causes of mild to moderate splenomegaly include infective endocarditis, which tends to run a subacute course in most cases. Systemic lupus erythematosus usually causes mild splenomegaly. Mild splenomegaly is common in infectious mononucleosis.

7-19   Correct answers (a), (c), (d), (e).
The word 'pancytopenia' means a reduction in cell numbers in all the haematological cell lines. These patients have anaemia and a low white cell count, and because of the latter an increased susceptibility to infection. Underlying malignancy (haematological or metastatic malignancy) affecting the bone marrow is a possible, but by no means the only cause. Myelofibrosis, hypersplenism, AIDS and vitamin B_{12} deficiency are other important causes.

7-20   Correct answers (a), (b), (c).
In acute leukaemia infection, bleeding, hepatomegaly and splenomegaly, lympha-denopathy (usually acute lymphocytic leukaemia) and bone pain are common features. Patients with acute leukemia may have infiltration of the spinal cord and nerve roots, and the tonsils. Atrophy of the spleen and an increased platelet count are not typical.

7-21   Correct answers (b), (d).
Patients with chronic renal failure tend to have a low erythropoietin level since the hormone is produced in the kidneys, probably in the peritubular interstitial cells in the inner cortex and outer medulla. Chronic hypoxia leads to increased release of erythropoietin and a compensating increase in the number of red blood cells. Patients with acyanotic congenital heart disease do not have significant hypoxia and these conditions are not associated with an increased erythropoietin level. Erythropoietin levels may be directly increased in patients with hepatocellular carcinoma. Erythropoietin tumours have not been described.

7-22   Correct answers (a), (b), (c), (d).
Renal impairment is common in patients with multiple myeloma (25%) for several possible reasons. Hypercalcaemia is the most common explanation but glomerular deposits (e.g. urate, amyloid, infection or rarely myeloma cell infiltration) or tubular

damage from light chains can also occur. Anaemia is very common in myeloma patients (80%). It is often due to replacement of normal marrow by tumour cells. Anaemia itself, however, is *not* a cause of renal impairment.

Chapter 8
The Rheumatological System

8-1   Both statements are true.
Arthralgia is joint pain without swelling.

8-2   Correct answers (a), (b). Reference: page 247.
Morning stiffness for over an hour is typical of an inflammatory arthritis but is not a feature of osteoarthritis. The more severe the joint disease the longer the morning stiffness tends to last. It can occur in any of the inflammatory arthritides. It is not in itself an indication for the use of steroids.

8-3   Correct answers (c), (d). Reference: page 248.
Rheumatoid arthritis more often presents with polyarthropathy. Infective arthritis is more often a monoarthritis. Monoarthritis can be a manifestation of gout or trauma. Pseudogout can also cause a monoarthritis.

8-4   Correct answers (b), (e). Reference: page 248.
Viral infection is not an uncommon cause of polyarthritis and destructive changes are very rare. Disseminated bacterial infection can cause polyarthritis and it can be a presenting feature of connective tissue disease.

8-5   Correct answers (a), (c), (d), (e). Reference: page 249.
Rheumatoid arthritis often affects the hands first. Ankylosing spondylitis characteristically involves the sacroiliac joints but these are not always the first to be affected. Psoriatic arthritis may typically affect the terminal interphalangeal joints. Other forms of psoriatic arthritis may mimic rheumatoid arthritis. Reiter's syndrome tends to affect the ankles and feet though it can also present with a clinical picture identical to ankylosing spondylitis.

8-6   Correct answer (d). Reference: page 255.
These fingers show the typical changes of osteoarthritis with Heberden's (distal interphalangeal) and Bouchard's (proximal interphalangeal) nodes.

8-7   Correct answers (a), (b), (c), (d). Reference: page 250.
Raynaud's phenomenon is the appearance of characteristic colour changes in the fingers (white, blue then red) in response to cold weather. The idiopathic form (Raynaud's disease) more often affects women. Drugs which cause peripheral vasoconstriction such as beta-blockers tend to make the condition worse. Raynaud's phenomenon can be secondary to rheumatoid arthritis or a connective tissue disease such as scleroderma.

8-8   Correct answers (a), (b), (c), (d). Reference: page 255.
This patient's hands show characteristic changes of rheumatoid arthritis except that pannus formation over the wrists is not visible.

8-9   Correct answers (b), (c), (d), (e). Reference: page 269.
The changes in the feet are typical of rheumatoid arthritis.

8-10   Correct answers (c), (d). Reference: page 276.
This patient's hands have very large gouty tophi which are packed full of urate crystals.

8-11   Correct answers (b), (c), (d).
This is the correct way of examining the hands of patients with suspected inflammatory arthritis. It is possible to test movement and assess tenderness at each of the joints of the hand in this way. Care should be taken not to hurt the patient but this is not usually a painful way to examine.

8-12   Both statements are false. Reference: page 262.
This patient has rheumatoid arthritis with rheumatoid nodules, not tendon xanthomata, present near the elbows.

8-13   Correct answers (b), (c), (d). Reference: page 281.
These hands show the changes of scleroderma with fixed flexion of the fingers. The skin is tethered on the dorsal surfaces of the hands and up on to the forearms. Restriction of mouth opening by tight skin on the face can be a problem. These patients often have oesophageal motility disorders and difficulty swallowing.

8-14   Correct answers (b), (d).
It is not possible to inspect the hip joint. Joint tenderness may be felt over the outer half of the inguinal ligament. Normal abduction is possible to about 50 degrees. Adduction is usually possible to 45 degrees. Rotation (external and internal) is tested with the knee and hip flexed.

8-15   Correct answers (a), (b), (c), (d). Reference: page 268.
Only a small amount of lateral movement of the leg on the knee joint is usually possible. Similarly, only small amounts of anterior and posterior movement of the leg on the knee are possible if the cruciate ligaments are normal. Quadriceps wasting, not hypertrophy, may occur with disease of the knee joint.

8-16   Correct answers (a), (c), (d), (e). Reference: page 270.
Sausage deformity of the fingers and toes is typical of psoriatic arthritis and Reiter's syndrome. Patients with psoriatic arthritis have associated pitting of the finger and toe nails. The typical rash appears on the extensor surfaces of the elbows and knees but may be hidden in the scalp, umbilicus or gluteal folds. In Reiter's syndrome, circinate balanitis is common. The rash is not pruritic.

8-17   Correct answers (d), (e). Reference: page 269.
The range of movement at the subtalar joint is limited, but tenderness on movement is an important sign.

8-18   Both statements are true. Reference: page 274.
Plantar fasciitis is characteristic of the seronegative spondyloarthropathies. It results in tenderness over the inferior aspect of the heel.

8-19   First statement true; second statement false. Reference: page 271.
Patients with rheumatoid arthritis may appear Cushingoid because of steroid treatment. Cushing's syndrome is not associated with rheumatoid arthritis.

8-20   Correct answers (a), (b), (e). Reference: page 273.
The typical eye changes in rheumatoid arthritis include episcleritis and signs of anaemia. Sjögren's syndrome is an association. Iritis does not occur.

8-21   Correct answers (a), (c). Reference: page 274.
Cardiac involvement in rheumatoid arthritis may include pericarditis leading to a pericardial rub. Occasionally, a rheumatoid nodule may affect the aortic valve and cause aortic regurgitation.

8-22   **Correct answers (a), (b), (c), (d), (e). Reference: page 274.**
All these changes are common in knees affected by rheumatoid arthritis. Rheumatoid nodules develop in 20–30% of rheumatoid arthritis patients, typically in areas subject to mechanical pressure, such as periarticular structures or extensor surfaces (but they can occur elsewhere).

8-23   **First statement true; second statement false. Reference: page 274.**
Foot drop may occur in patients with rheumatoid arthritis because of nerve entrapment. Lumbar disc disease is not a feature of rheumatoid arthritis.

8-24   **Correct answer (d). Reference: page 274.**
Mixed connective tissue disease is not one of the seronegative spondyloarthropathies.

8-25   **Correct answers (a), (b), (d). Reference: page 275.**
Reiter's syndrome is one of the seronegative spondyloarthropathies. There is a characteristic rash of the glans penis and conjunctivitis. Painless mouth ulcers may be present. The wrist joints may be involved if the arthritis follows a rheumatoid pattern but nodules do not occur.

8-26   **Correct answers (b), (d). Reference: page 276.**
Enteropathic arthritis can be associated with either ulcerative colitis or Crohn's disease. One form involves the peripheral joints, usually in an asymmetrical pattern. The other is very similar to ankylosing spondylitis. Joint deformity is not common.

8-27   **Correct answer (e). Reference: page 276.**
Gout can affect many parts of the body but not usually the costochondral junctions.

8-28   **Correct answer (d). Reference: page 277.**
Systemic lupus erythematosus (SLE) is not associated with rheumatoid nodules. Patients can develop psychosis because of steroid treatment or from the condition itself because of cerebral vasculitis. Photosensitivity rashes and Raynaud's phenomenon are common. Occasionally arthritis in a rheumatoid pattern may appear.

8-29   **Correct answers (a), (b), (e). Reference: page 279.**
Short broken hairs present over the forehead are typical of SLE; these are called lupus hairs. Patchy alopecia is common. Hair changes similar to those in hypothyroidism may occur: the hair becomes coarse and dry.

8-30   **Correct answer (d). Reference: page 279.**
There are a number of eye changes common in patients with SLE but lens dislocation is not one of them.

8-31   **Correct (b), (c), (d). Reference: page 281.**
Patients with scleroderma tend to lose weight. The skin becomes indurated, and non-pitting oedema may be present; this occurs especially in the hands and forearms. The deposition of calcium in the subcutaneous tissues (calcinosis) is typical of scleroderma or the CREST syndrome (calcinosis, Raynaud's phenomenon, oesophageal dysmotility, sclerodactyly and telangiectasia). Raynaud's phenomenon is common in scleroderma.

8-32   **Correct answers (a), (c), (d), (e). Reference: page 284.**
The major criteria for the diagnosis include polyarthritis, signs of pancarditis, the presence of Sydenham's chorea (which is very rare and is characterised by non-repetitive, abrupt involuntary jerks of the limbs) and subcutaneous nodules. A red throat is not a major or minor criterion for rheumatic fever.

Chapter 9
The Endocrine System

9-1 **Correct answer (a). Reference: page 292, 293.**
Male and female patterns of hair distribution on the body have a hormonal basis. Androgen excess in women causes a male pattern of hair distribution and androgen deficiency in men causes loss of male body hair. Although tall stature (growth hormone excess in childhood (gigantism)), headache (pituitary tumours and acromegaly), male baldness, sweatiness (acromegaly) and obesity (Cushing's syndrome) may be caused by endocrine excesses of various sorts, these conditions are very common and are not usually related to endocrine disease.

9-2 **Correct answers (a), (b), (c). Reference: page 292.**
Many patients complain of weight gain, but the most common cause is probably overeating. Hypothyroid patients put on weight (reduced metabolic rate) as do those with Cushing's syndrome (a result of steroid excess and partly due to an associated increased appetite). Uncontrolled diabetics tend to lose weight (anorexia and loss of glucose and ketones) and patients with advanced malignant disease also usually lose weight (a combination of anorexia and release of tumour factors).

9-3 **Correct answers (a), (b), (c), (e). Reference: page 308.**
The acral parts of the body are the hands and feet which become larger in adult patients with acromegaly. Once epiphyseal closure has occurred, growth of long bones is not possible but thickening of the ends of bones and of soft tissues can continue. Facial features also coarsen, the tongue enlarges and there is wide spacing of the teeth. Characteristically, patients who wear hats notice an increase in hat size. The voice deepens and becomes more hollow because of enlargement of the larynx and sinuses.

9-4 **Correct answer (a). Reference: page 320.**
The symptoms of diabetes mellitus vary. Patients may present with blurred vision (due to changes in lens hydration), mucosal and skin infections (because of hyperglycaemia) and generalised weakness (a combination of reduction in cell uptake of glucose and dehydration caused by glucose-induced diuresis). Appetite tends to increase, but seriously ill patients with ketoacidosis may have anorexia.

9-5 **Correct answers (b), (c). Reference: page 293.**
Thyrotoxic patients usually feel rather energetic probably as a result of increased metabolic activity. Uncontrolled diabetes mellitus induces lethargy, as does inadequate cortisol secretion because of adrenal failure. Patients with a phaeochromocytoma may present with palpitations and hypertension (due to adrenaline and noradrenaline secretion by the tumour), but not usually with tiredness. Hyperinsulinaemia is rare, but presents with dizziness and syncope (due to hypoglycaemia caused by autonomous insulin secretion) rather than with lethargy.

9-6 **Correct answer (d). Reference: page 293.**
Skin tags are associated with acromegaly. Increased skin pigmentation occurs in Addison's disease because of increased ACTH secretion (ACTH has melanocyte-stimulating activity). Flushing of the face and neck may rarely be due to carcinoid syndrome (these gastrointestinal endocrine tumours secrete, among other substances, serotonin which is responsible for cutaneous flushing). Scattered areas of skin atrophy are not typical of any endocrine condition. Acanthosis nigricans, which is a furry black discoloration in the axillae, can be associated with acromegaly.

9-7 **Correct answers (a), (b), (c), (e). Reference: page 294, 315.**
Most short people merely have short parents, although all but one of the endocrine diseases listed in the question can rarely cause short stature. Childhood growth hor-

mone deficiency should be considered for children more than three standard deviations below the predicted height for age. Systemic disease, hypothyroidism and chromosomal disorders may cause short stature. Klinefelter's syndrome is a chromosomal disorder (XXY) usually associated with tall stature.

9-8   Correct answer (a). Reference: page 294.
There are many causes of male impotence including vascular disease involving the pelvic arteries, diabetes mellitus, hypogonadism, hyperprolactinaemia and haemochromatosis, but the most common cause is psychological dysfunction.

9-9   Correct answers (c), (d), (e). Reference: page 294.
If menstruation has not begun by the age of 17 years, primary amenorrhoea is diagnosed. Systemic diseases including chronic renal failure and malabsorption are more common causes than endocrine disease. Psychiatric disease, particularly anorexia nervosa, can be a cause.

9-10   Correct answers (a), (d). Reference: page 294.
Urinary frequency is different from polyuria. Patients may pass frequent small amounts of urine because of bladder irritability; this is termed urinary frequency. A patient who passes more than three litres of urine a day is considered to have polyuria. Both diabetes mellitus and diabetes insipidus can cause polyuria. The word 'diabetes' means increased urine flow. Compulsive water drinking is a well-known cause of polyuria. In some forms of renal failure, larger than normal amounts of urine are produced because the kidneys are unable to concentrate urine normally.

9-11   Correct answer (e). Reference: page 295.
Mothers with diabetes mellitus often have a history of giving birth to a large baby before the diabetes was diagnosed. Carcinoma of the lung has been shown to be responsible for numerous endocrine abnormalities because of hormone production by the neoplasm. Skin and foot infections are common in diabetics and may present before the disease is diagnosed. Patients with thyroid disease may have had a previous partial or complete thyroidectomy, while patients with parathyroid disease may have had a neck exploration. Unexplained weight gain may be due to endocrine disease (e.g. Cushing's syndrome) but this is not the most common cause.

9-12   Correct answers (b), (c). Reference: page 295.
Diabetic patients must be responsible for the day-to-day management of their condition. Many may understand the difference between human and animal insulin. This is not likely to make a big difference to their day-to-day treatment. Patients should know their current insulin dose and be well aware of symptoms suggesting hypoglycaemia. Patients should at least be able to test their urine for sugar, and most these days should be able to test their blood sugar level. Patients should be aware of the need to seek medical help when their blood sugars are very high, but cannot be expected to know how to treat diabetic ketoacidosis.

9-13   Correct answers (b), (d). Reference: page 295.
Hypoadrenalism is a chronic condition and the patient should have some understanding of the treatment. Patients need not make adjustments to their own steroid doses at times of anxiety, but must be advised to inform medical attendants of their condition so that increased steroid doses can be given at times of physical stress, such as surgical operations. Steroid doses are not adjusted to take into account day-to-day activity. An explanation of the role of steroids is important for the patient. Testing of blood levels is not relevant on a day-to-day basis and is not performed by the patient.

9-14   Correct answer (c). Reference: page 296.
The normal thyroid gland can sometimes be felt in thin patients but should not descend into the chest. Large goitres are usually obvious on inspection, but the thyroid gland can

be felt to move upwards during swallowing, not down. Enlarged thyroids are not usually tender unless thyroiditis is present.

9-15   Correct answers (a), (b), (e). Reference: page 296.
An enlarged thyroid has a fairly typical appearance but can occasionally be confused with a thyroglossal cyst or large lymph nodes (e.g. with a lymphoma). The carotid artery is normally placed laterally and can be felt to pulsate. The trachea, composed partly of cartilage, feels quite different from the thyroid.

9-16   Correct answer (d). Reference: page 299.
The fingernail in this photograph shows onycholysis. There is separation of the distal part of the nail from the nail bed. This condition can be associated with thyrotoxicosis.

9-17   Correct answer (a), (e). Reference: page 302.
This patient looks hypothyroid. Apathy is often a feature of this condition. Weight gain is also common. The reflexes are usually reduced or 'hung up'. The heart rate is typically slow. Coarse, croaking slow speech is typical. Spade-like hands occur as a result of acral enlargement (acromegaly).

9-18   Correct answers (a), (b), (c), (d). Reference: page 308.
This patient looks acromegalic. The changes of acromegaly are very gradual and they may not be noticed by patients or their relatives. An increase in hat size is sometimes noticed by those who wear hats. Macroglossia or enlargement of the tongue is often present. The hands tend to become very large. There is usually proximal muscle weakness. The enlarging pituitary tumour which causes the condition results typically in a bitemporal hemianopia, but other types of field loss may also occur.

9-19   Correct answers (a), (b), (c). Reference: page 319.
This man has gynaecomastia. It should be distinguished from the presence of adipose tissue (lipomastia). This unusual enlargement of the breasts in men has a number of causes including testicular failure (e.g. tumour, orchitis), chronic liver disease, thyrotoxicosis, carcinoma (e.g. lung, adrenal) and the use of certain drugs including spironolactone and cimetidine. The presence of abdominal distension (and probable ascites) suggests chronic liver disease in this case. The condition occurs when the normal male ratio of oestrogen to androgen rises. This may be a result of reduction in testosterone production or increased oestrogen production. Spironolactone and cimetidine appear to block androgen binding.

9-20   Correct answers (b), (d), (e). Reference: page 313.
These hands show vitiligo. This is a localised depigmentation which can involve any part of the body. It may be associated with autoimmune adrenal failure, pernicious anaemia and autoimmune thyroid disease (the autoimmune cluster).

9-21   Correct answers (b), (c), (d). Reference: page 315.
This patient's hands have short fourth and fifth fingers. This is characteristic of pseudo-hypoparathyroidism (type Ia) and pseudopseudohypoparathyroidism. The former patients have a tissue resistance to the effects of parathyroid hormone and may have symptoms and signs of hypocalcaemia. The toes may be short in the same way as the fingers. The patients are usually of short stature.

9-22   Correct answers (b), (d), (e). Reference: page 318.
An increase in facial and body hair (hirsutism) is a common worry for women, but is often normal. If there are signs of virilisation, this strongly suggests an endocrine abnormality. Polycystic ovaries can cause hirsutism. Virilising drugs are an occasional cause.

9-23 **Correct answers (a), (c), (e). Reference: page 317.**
People with Down's syndrome have an increased risk of certain cardiac defects. These include atrial and ventricular septal defects. Coding for the formation of the atrioventricular canal in embryonic development appears to be on chromosome 21. Down's syndrome usually involves trisomy 21. They characteristically have short broad hands and oblique orbital fissures. The palate may be high and broad.

9-24 **Correct answers (c), (e).**
Proliferative retinal changes are more likely to cause retinal damage and interfere with vision than non-proliferative changes. Not all diabetics have haemorrhages in their eyes. The treatment of proliferative changes includes laser therapy which leaves small scars on the retina. The new vessel formation characteristic of proliferative change is damaging to the retina. It can result in retinal detachment and blindness.

9-25 **Correct answers (c), (d), (e). Reference: page 326.**
Paget's disease of bone is due to increased osteoclast activity. It can cause limb deformity and may be of viral origin. There is an increased risk of the development of sarcoma. Oddly enough, bronchial breath sounds may be heard if one listens over the skull with the stethoscope.

9-26 **Correct answers (a), (b), (d). Reference: page 326.**
Angioid streaks in the fundi may occur in patients with Paget's disease as well as in those with acromegaly. The eighth nerve may become trapped and the ossicles may be abnormal in Paget's disease; either or both of these problems can cause deafness. Anosmia is not a usual feature, but the cranial nerves may be affected by overgrowth of their foramina in Paget's disease. Women and men are both affected.

9-27 **Both statements are true. Reference: page 313.**
Patients with Addison's disease may become hyperpigmented because of the melanocyte stimulating activity present in ACTH.

9-28 **First statement true; second statement false. Reference: page 312.**
One should palpate the abdomen of a patient with Cushing's syndrome, but large adrenal carcinomas are a very rare cause of this condition.

9-29 **Both statements are false. Reference: page 309.**
Patients with acromegaly have small testes because of reduced secretion of pituitary hormones. Enlargement of a growth hormone secreting tumour eventually compresses and damages gonadotrophin secreting cells in the pituitary.

Chapter 10
The Nervous System

10-1 **Correct answer (a).**
There are many causes of headache, and careful history-taking will usually allow a correct diagnosis to be made. Tension headaches are commonly bilateral, occur over the frontal or temporal areas and typically are described as a tightness; these headaches can last for hours and recur often. Migraine is usually a throbbing hemicranial headache accompanied by nausea and vomiting; classic migraine begins with a prodrome (e.g. dazzling zigzag lines, visual scintillations, photophobia) but common migraine has no prodrome. Cluster headaches are constant unilateral pain over the orbit recurring nightly for a period and associated with rhinorrhoea and ipsilateral Horner's syndrome. Raised intracranial pressure, from a tumour for example, will often cause projectile

vomiting. The headache of a brain tumour will not have been present for years, tends to be recurrent daily and may often wake the patient from sleep. Photophobia and fever as well as neck stiffness suggest meningitis.

10-2   Correct answer (b).
Neck stiffness is an important sign and should be tested for as part of the neurological examination. In a febrile patient, the possibility of meningitis always needs to be considered; neck stiffness would indicate the need for lumbar puncture to determine if this is the correct diagnosis. Neck stiffness does not occur in cerebrovascular disease unless there is a subarachnoid haemorrhage. Neck stiffness is not a sign of raised intracranial pressure. Higher centre disorders cause difficulties with orientation, speech and other higher functions, but not neck stiffness.

10-3   Correct answer 3(a), 2(b), 1(c).
Listening to a patient's speech can give a diagnosis. It is important to distinguish dysarthria (or difficulty with articulation) from dysphasia (a disorder in the use of the symbols of communication due to a dominant higher centre disease process). Disorganised fluent speech in a patient who has trouble understanding commands suggests a receptive (or posterior) dysphasia, which occurs with a lesion of the dominant hemisphere in the posterior part of the first temporal gyrus (Wernicke's area). Slurred speech occurs with dysarthria and is the typical finding in intoxicated individuals. Patients who are unable to name objects but otherwise have normal speech have nominal dysphasia, which can be caused by a lesion of the dominant posterior temporoparietal area.

10-4   Correct answers (b), (c), (d), (e).
Examination of the visual fields is part of the cranial nerve examination of the second (optic) nerve. A bitemporal hemianopia occurs with a lesion of the optic chiasm such as a pituitary tumour or a sella meningioma. Parietal lobe lesions do not produce a bitemporal hemianopia. Papilloedema can produce peripheral constriction of the visual fields, as can glaucoma. A temporal lobe lesion can produce a homonymous hemianopia or superior quadrantanopia. A lesion of the optic nerve or disease in this area can produce unilateral field loss. The blind spot is a small area close to the centre of the visual fields where there is no vision; this represents the area where the optic disc is seen on fundoscopy and is the point where the optic nerve joins the retina. This spot can be mapped and is enlarged in patients with papilloedema when there is swelling of the optic disc.

10-5   Correct answers (a), (b), (c), (e).
Fundal haemorrhages seen on fundoscopy include linear or flame shaped haemorrhages near the vessels, large ecchymoses that obliterate vessels, petechiae which may be confused with microaneurysms and subhyaloid haemorrhages. Linear haemorrhages and ecchymoses occur in hypertension or diabetic retinopathy. Raised intracranial pressure and bleeding diatheses may also produce these haemorrhages. Petechiae occur in diabetes mellitus. Subhyaloid haemorrhages are seen with subarachnoid haemorrhage. Retinitis pigmentosa manifests as a scattering of black retinal pigment in a crisscross pattern; it represents a form of retinal dystrophy that produces loss of peripheral vision and night blindness but does not cause haemorrhages.

10-6   Correct answers (b), (d).
When examining the pupils, testing the light reflex with a pocket torch is important. Normally the pupil constricts briskly in direct response to light while the opposite pupil also constricts (the consensual response). If the torch is moved in an arc from pupil to pupil, and there is severely reduced visual acuity from optic nerve disease such as optic atrophy, the affected pupil will paradoxically dilate after a short time when the torch is moved from the normal eye to the abnormal eye; this is called the Marcus Gunn or afferent pupillary defect. It is not a sign of hysteria. Argyll-Robertson pupils on the

other hand refer to the absence of the light reflex but an intact accommodation reflex, which can occur with a midbrain lesion (e.g. in syphilis).

10-7   Correct answers (a), (b), (c), (d), (e).
Nystagmus results from disturbances of the balance of tone between opposing ocular muscles, allowing the eyes to drift in one direction which is then corrected by a quick (saccadic) movement back to the original position. Drugs such as alcohol or phenytoin, vestibular lesions and brainstem disease can all cause jerky nystagmus. Decreased macular vision causes pendular nystagmus.

10-8   Correct answer (d).
The corneal reflex is mediated by the ophthalmic division of the V cranial nerve for the sensory component and the VII (facial) nerve for the reflex blink motor response of the orbicularis oculi muscle. Therefore, if a corneal reflex is elicited, this tests two cranial nerves and indicates that these tracts are normal. The corneal reflex does not assess macular vision, hearing (VIII nerve) or cerebellar function.

10-9   Correct answer (c).
Causes of a supranuclear facial palsy (upper motor neurone lesion) include vascular lesions or tumours. Bell's palsy (an idiopathic acute paralysis of the nerve) is the most common cause of a lower motor neurone VII nerve lesion. Bell's phenomenon is the upward movement of the eyeball with incomplete closure of the eyelid that can be seen with facial weakness of any aetiology. The forehead muscles are preserved on the side of an upper motor neurone lesion because of bilateral cortical representation of these muscles. Drooping of the corner of the mouth typically occurs with an upper motor neurone lesion affecting the facial nerve. The facial nerve does not supply sensation and therefore there is no loss of sensation on the affected side.

10-10   Correct answer (a).
Testing hearing is useful. If abnormal, evidence of nerve and conduction deafness should be evaluated by Rinné's and Weber's tests. Rinné's test is described in this question. With nerve deafness, the note remains audible at the external meatus as air and bone conduction are reduced equally so that air conduction is better (as is normal). Therefore, the test suggests nerve deafness in this patient. Wax in the ear can cause conduction deafness, as can otitis media, but the normal Rinné's test does not suggest there is conduction deafness.

10-11   Correct answer (a).
The gag reflex tests the IX cranial nerve (sensory component) and the X cranial nerve (motor component). Absence of the gag reflex may indicate a lower motor neurone lesion of IX. The gag reflex is not affected by the other cranial nerves listed in the question.

10-12   Correct answers (a), (b).
The examiner in Photograph 10.1 is testing the supinator (brachioradialis) jerk. This involves striking the lower end of the radius above the wrist and watching for flexion of the elbow and contraction of the brachioradialis. This tests the segmental innervation of C5–C6, not C8. Elbow extension will occur only if there is a lesion within the spinal canal causing damage to C5–C6 nerve roots and the adjacent spinal cord ('inverted supinator reflex'). Finger jerks (C8) are elicited by striking the examiner's fingers, that are in turn interlocked over the patient's, and looking for slight flexion of all the fingers.

10-13   Correct answers (c), (e).
Inspecting the large muscles for irregular non-rhythmical contractions (fasciculations) is very important. These may be fine or coarse, and are most easily seen in the deltoid and calf muscles. Fasciculations are classically found in patients with motor neurone disease.

However, fasciculations alone do not make a diagnosis of motor neurone disease as there are other causes (although if there is fasciculation of the tongue and the jaw jerk is exaggerated, this usually indicates that motor neurone disease is the correct diagnosis). In thyrotoxic myopathy, the muscles are usually wasted, reflexes are reduced and fasciculations may be seen. Fasciculations may also occur in rare forms of myositis, with motor root compression or in peripheral neuropathies. Fasciculations are usually benign if there is no associated weakness and wasting of the muscles. Tapping over the muscles to elicit fasciculations is no longer considered to be clinically useful because contractions stimulated by tapping do not indicate that fasciculations are present. Horner's syndrome refers to interruption of the sympathetic innervation of the eye at any point resulting in partial ptosis, a constricted pupil and sometimes decreased facial sweating; it has nothing to do with fasciculations.

10-14   Correct answers (a), (b), (c), (d), (e).
The planter reflex is useful for looking for evidence of an upper motor neurone (pyramidal) lesion. A sharp, but not too sharp, object is stroked up the lateral aspect of the sole, curving inwards before it reaches the toes to move towards the middle metatarsophalangeal joint. Normally, in an adult, there is flexion of the big toe at the metatarsophalangeal joint. Extension of the big toe (an upgoing toe or a positive Babinski's sign) indicates an upper motor neurone lesion which can be caused by disease interrupting the neural pathways at any level above the anterior horn cell, including cerebrovascular accidents (strokes) and spinal cord disease. Bilateral upgoing toes may occur in coma or after generalised seizures.

10-15   Correct answer (a).
Drifting of the arms with the eyes closed can be caused by one of three conditions: upper motor neurone weakness, which tends to lead to drifting in a downward direction; cerebellar disease, where hypotonia usually causes upward drifting of the arms; and loss of proprioception. One would not expect a left cerebellar hemisphere lesion to cause right arm drift (the signs occur on the same side as a cerebellar lesion). Loss of proprioception may occur with cervical spondylosis and posterior compression of the cervical cord, although in such cases both arms are usually affected. Other causes of proprioceptive loss include tabes dorsalis and sensory neuropathy (e.g. from a carcinoma) which may affect the arms and legs. Fasciculations are irregular contractions of small areas of muscle with no rhythmical pattern; they are not related to drifting of the arm.

10-16   Correct answers (b), (d), (e).
Carefully observing the patient walking is part of the neurological examination. In hemiplegia, the foot is typically plantar flexed and the leg is swung out in a wide lateral arc. Common peroneal nerve palsy causes footdrop, but in this situation the gait is high stepping. In Parkinson's disease a shuffling gait, with difficulty starting and stopping and lack of an arm swing, is typical. A waddling gait is typical of proximal myopathy and not hemiplegia. Disease of the posterior columns can occur with subacute combined degeneration of the cord in Vitamin B_{12} deficiency. Posterior column lesions typically produce a gait with clumsy slapping down of the feet on a broad base. Finally, a prefrontal lobe lesion can produce a gait where the feet appear to be glued to the floor when the patient is erect but move more easily when the patient is lying down.

10-17   Correct answer (a).
Hemisection of the spinal cord (the Brown-Séquard syndrome) causes motor and sensory changes. The motor changes involve upper motor neurone signs below the hemisection on the same side as the lesion, and lower motor neurone signs at the level of the hemisection on the same side as the lesion. Vibration and proprioceptive loss occur on the same side as the lesion, but pain and temperature loss occur on the

opposite side to the lesion. With a spinal cord lesion, there is no sensory loss over the face. In the lateral medullary syndrome, pain and temperature loss occurs over the side of the face ipsilateral to the lesion and over the opposite side of the trunk and limbs.

10-18   Correct answers (a), (b), (c), (d), (e).
Inability to let go of the hand when shaking hands suggests myotonia. Patients with dystrophia myotonica characteristically have frontal baldness, an expressionless triangular face, atrophy of the temporalis and masseter muscles, and partial ptosis. Testing for percussion myotonia by tapping over the thenar eminence is helpful for confirming the presence of myotonia. Testicular atrophy, wasting and weakness of the forearm, hand and calf muscles, gynaecomastia, cardiac conduction abnormalities and cardiac failure from cardiomyopathy may be present. This disease is associated with diabetes mellitus and hence there may be sugar in the urine.

10-19   Correct answers (a), (c), (d), (e).
The ulnar nerve usually supplies all the small muscles of the hand except for the lateral two lumbricals, the opponens pollicis, the abductor pollicis brevis and the flexor pollicis brevis (the LOAF muscles are supplied by the median nerve). Partial clawing of the hand, with hyperextension at the metacarpophalangeal joints and flexion of the interphalangeal joints, occurs with an ulnar nerve lesion at the wrist (a more proximal ulnar nerve lesion causes less clawing because of the loss of flexor digitorum profundus function). Sensory loss occurs over the palmar and dorsal aspects of the little finger and medial half of the ring finger, not over the thumb. Wrist drop does not occur with an ulnar nerve lesion, but does occur with a radial nerve lesion. Abduction of the thumb (a function of the abductor pollicis brevis) is intact with an ulnar nerve lesion but not with a median nerve lesion (this can be tested by placing a pen over the laid-out hand of the patient, palm upward, and asking the patient to attempt to abduct the thumb vertically to touch the examiner's pen).

10-20   Correct answer (a), (b), (e).
Tremor may be due to Parkinson's disease; classically it occurs at rest. Action tremors occur throughout movement but resolve at rest and can be caused by thyrotoxicosis or drugs. Intention tremors in cerebellar disease increase as the hand moves towards the target. Chorea on the other hand refers to non-repetitive, abrupt involuntary jerky movements that should not be confused with tremor. This occurs in Huntington's disease as well as in other conditions (e.g. Wilson's disease or with drugs). Dystonia refers to an involuntary abnormal posture with excessive co-contraction of antagonist muscles.

10-21   Correct answer (c).
As part of the optic nerve examination, the visual fields should be tested by confrontation using a hat pin or the examiner's fingers. A lesion of the optic chiasm (site 5) causes a bitemporal hemianopia because the lesion damages fibres from the nasal halves of the retinas as they decussate, resulting in loss of both temporal halves of the visual fields. Bitemporal hemianopia may be due to a pituitary tumour, craniopharyngioma or a suprasellar meningioma.

10-22   Correct answer (a).
Interruption of the optic tract after the optic chiasm produces an homonymous hemianopia. In the optic tract the defect is typically complete and there is no macular sparing. Common causes include a vascular lesion or a cerebral tumour. Loss of central (macular) vision alone indicates that the lesion is anterior to the chiasm. This is most often due to senile macular degeneration (a macular hole) but can also occur in multiple sclerosis. Unilateral field loss indicates an optic nerve lesion or local eye disease. Concentric diminution of a field (tunnel vision) may be due to glaucoma or retinal abnormalities such as chorioretinitis or retinitis pigmentosa, as well as papilloedema.

10-23　Correct answer (d).

The pen touching test assesses the abductor pollicis brevis, a muscle supplied by the median nerve. The patient is asked to lay his or her hand flat with the palm upward on the table and attempt to abduct the thumb vertically to touch the examiner's pen held above it. This is not possible if there is a median nerve palsy at the wrist or above. As the patient successfully performed the test in Photograph 10.4, one can conclude that the median nerve is likely to be intact. Sensory loss in the median nerve distribution (the palmar aspect of the thumb, index, middle and lateral half of the ring fingers) is also likely to be intact. Neither ulnar nor radial nerve function is assessed by the pen touching test.

10-24　Correct answers (a), (d).

Figure 10.5 shows a partial left ptosis and meiosis, which occur in Horner's syndrome. Here there is interruption of the sympathetic innervation of the eye at some point. Horner's syndrome can occur as part of the lateral medullary syndrome in patients with a stroke. In this syndrome, Horner's syndrome occurs with nystagmus to the side of the lesion, ipsilateral pain and temperature loss over the face, as well as signs of a IX and X cranial nerve lesion, ipsilateral cerebellar signs, and contralateral pain and temperature loss over the trunk and limbs. Horner's syndrome is associated with decreased sweating over the affected eyebrow. Exophthalmos does not occur in Horner's syndrome; enophthalmos, or retraction of the eye, while often mentioned as a feature of Horner's syndrome, probably does not occur in man. It is important to examine the respiratory system, as carcinoma of the apex of the lung (usually a squamous cell carcinoma) can cause Horner's syndrome. Myasthenia gravis is an autoimmune disease of the neuromuscular junction which may cause unilateral or bilateral ptosis, particularly if the patient is asked to maintain a sustained upward gaze. Myasthenia gravis does not cause a constricted pupil.

10-25　Correct answers (a), (b), (c), (d), (e).

It is important to memorise the dermatomes to help one interpret sensory signs. It is useful to try to fit the distribution of any sensory loss into a dermatomal, single peripheral nerve, peripheral neuropathy (glove and stocking) or hemisensory pattern to determine the likely site and type of lesion.

10-26　Correct answers (b), (d).

When testing tone in the upper limb, flexion and extension of the wrist and elbow joint should be performed passively. It is important to decide if tone is normal, increased or decreased. Increased tone occurs with upper motor neurone lesions or extrapyramidal lesions. Therefore, Parkinson's syndrome (extrapyramidal diseases) and hemiplegia (from an upper motor neurone lesion) will cause hypertonia. On the other hand, lower motor neurone lesions cause hypotonia. Mononeuritis multiplex refers to separate involvement of more than one peripheral (or rarely cranial) nerve. This can be caused acutely by diabetes mellitus or polyarteritis nodosa, or chronically by multiple compressive neuropathies, sarcoidosis, acromegaly, leprosy and rarely carcinoma.

10-27　Correct answers (a), (b).

The signs described in this 30-year-old patient are upper motor neurone signs in the lower limbs, with typical weakness without wasting, hypertonia and clonus, and an extensor plantar response. However, it is important to note that the knee and ankle reflexes are absent rather than increased, as would be expected with an upper motor neurone lesion. This suggests that there is a combination of upper and lower motor neurone signs in this case. In addition, there is selective posterior column loss symmetrically, with absence of vibration and joint position sense. Dissociated sensory (in this case posterior column) loss without spinothalamic (pain and temperature) loss usually suggests spinal cord disease, although dissociation can occur with peripheral neuropathies. These signs can occur with subacute combined degeneration of the spinal cord. Vitamin B_{12} deficiency can cause subacute combined degeneration of the cord and, in this woman with long-standing terminal ileal disease, B_{12} malabsorption is likely to have occurred. Motor neurone disease can cause an extensor plantar response plus absent knee and ankle jerks, but dissociated sensory loss (and indeed objective sensory changes) would not be expected with motor neurone disease. Friedreich's ataxia is an autosomal recessive condition that can present in young persons with bilateral cerebellar signs, pes cavus, posterior column sensory loss in the limbs, and upper motor neurone signs in the limbs with absent ankle and knee reflexes due to peripheral neuropathy. Patients with Friedreich's ataxia may also have optic atrophy, cardiomyopathy and diabetes mellitus.

10-28   Correct answers (a), (b), (c), (d), (e).
When examining patients who complain of clumsiness or difficulty with coordination, it is important to assess for underlying cerebellar disease. Signs of cerebellar disease occur on the same side as the lesion in the brain. Signs to look for include nystagmus, cerebellar speech (which is typically jerky, explosive and loud with an irregular separation of syllables), and signs in the limbs including intention tremor (which increases as the target is approached), past-pointing (where the patient overshoots the target), an inability to perform rapidly alternating movements smoothly, truncal ataxia, and a 'drunken' gait that is wide-based, or reeling on a narrow base.

10-29   Correct answer (a).
Doll's eye testing is performed by lifting the patient's eyelids and rolling the head from side to side. When the vestibular reflexes are intact, indicating an intact brainstem, the eyes maintain their fixation as if looking at an object in the distance, although they change their position relative to the head; this is the normal doll's eye phenomenon. When the eyes move with the head so that fixation is not maintained, this suggests that there is a brainstem lesion or that drugs are affecting the brainstem. When the eyes both deviate to one side in a comatose patient, this may indicate a destructive lesion in the cerebral hemisphere ipsilaterally; this is not the doll's eye phenomenon. The cranial nerves can be assessed in part in a comatose patient by careful examination.

10-30   Both statements are correct.
Hypoglycaemia is a very important cause of coma because it is reversible. You should always consider this possibility whenever assessing a patient with an acute neurological disease.

10-31   Correct answers (b), (c), (d).
Idiopathic trigeminal neuralgia causes severe facial pain. It is not associated with sensory loss unless due to a posterior fossa mass. Temporal arteritis must always be considered a possible cause of headache in elderly people. Prompt treatment may prevent blindness. Intracranial pressure rises in the supine position and the headache that comes with it may be worse when the patient lies down. Unlike migraine, cluster headache is more common in men. An aneurysm on the posterior communicating artery can compress the oculomotor (III) nerve.

10-32   Correct answers (a), (c), (d), (e).
Ataxia and nystagmus are cerebellar signs. Phenytoin toxicity is a common and reversible cause. The other causes are usually conditions affecting the posterior fossa.

10-33   Correct answers (a), (c), (e).
The 'pill-rolling' resting tremor is characteristic of Parkinson's disease. Upper motor neurone signs are not a feature. Tone is abnormal (cogwheel rigidity) but not increased in an upper motor neurone 'clasp-knife' fashion. Changes in the substantia nigra are usually seen at autopsy, with a reduction in the number of dopaminergic neurones. Some cases of parkinsonism have occurred after viral epidemics; carbon monoxide poisoning, drugs and tumour are also uncommon causes.

10-34   Correct answers (a), (c).

Recurrent episodes of aphasia suggest a left cerebral embolic event involving the middle cerebral artery. This can be a result of left carotid artery disease. In this case emboli may also reach the left optic fundus where their effects can be seen on fundoscopy. Atrial fibrillation, especially if a patient has mitral stenosis, is an important precursor of cerebral embolic events.

10-35   Correct answers (d), (e).

Urinary incontinence does not occur early, and sudden changes are uncommon in patients with Alzheimer's disease.

10-36   Correct answer (a).

Common peroneal nerve palsy, unlike the other conditions listed, causes foot drop with sensory loss as described in this case. An L5 (butnot L3) root lesion can sometimes cause confusion but other signs are usually present (e.g. loss of the ankle jerk and L5 sensory loss). Amyotrophic lateral sclerosis (progressive motor neurone disease) is not associated with sensory changes of this type. Both multiple sclerosis and a right-sided internal capsular stroke could conceivably present in this way.

10-37   Correct answers (a), (d), (e).

Constructional and dressing apraxia are non-dominant parietal lobe signs. No conclusion as to the patient's handedness can be drawn from this. Visual inattention and agraphaesthesia (the inability to recognise numbers drawn on the skin) occur with parietal lesions on either side. The signs are present on the side opposite the lesion.

10-38   Correct answers (a), (b).

This drawing suggests that the patient has spatial neglect. It is more common with non-dominant parietal lesions. Dressing apraxia is usually present but anosmia is not related. Dysphasia suggests a dominant hemisphere lesion.

10-39   Correct answers (a), (d).

Since papilloedema is not due to primary disease of the optic nerve, visual acuity is preserved. Eye movement may cause discomfort in patients with inflammation of the optic nerve and therefore suggests papillitis. Papilloedema results from a rise in intracranial pressure and therefore tends to be bilateral. Papillitis is more often unilateral at first. The rapid onset of diminution of vision in the affected eye is a feature of papillitis.

10-40   Correct answers (c), (e).

A dilated pupil and complete ptosis occur with a third (III) nerve lesion. The pupillary response to light and accommodation is lost with a third nerve palsy and there are divergent visual axes — the eye is turned 'down and out'.

Chapter 11
The Psychiatric History And Mental State Examination

11-1   Correct answer (b).

The most important thing to do at the start of a psychiatric interview is to establish rapport with the patient, who will then be more willing to tell you about his or her difficulties. Orientation is generally tested towards the end of the interview when one is completing the cognitive tests of the mental state examination. A diagnosis and treatment plan is made for the patient at the end of the interview when the clinician has drawn together all of the information. Giving advice is not something usually done in an initial psychiatric interview.

11-2   **Correct answer (c).**
Echolalia is a phenomenon where the patient repeats words that have been said by the interviewer. Perceptual disturbances are part of all the other phenomena.

11-3   **Correct answer (d).**
This is a simple test of judgment. It assesses whether the patient would behave appropriately in this situation. Intelligence may contribute to a person's response to this, but it is not directly a test of intelligence. Abstract thinking is usually tested by asking the patient to interpret a proverb. Insight is judged during the course of the interview by assessing whether the patient considers himself or herself to be ill. Cognition is tested using the routine cognitive tests of the mental state examination.

11-4   **Correct answer (a).**
A stress interview, which may be appropriate in certain circumstances, will not improve rapport as it will make the patient feel anxious. Asking open-ended questions, however, helps because it encourages the patient to speak freely. Using the patient's words also helps the patient to feel understood. If the patient feels understood by the clinician, empathy will be improved. Uncovering the patient's feelings will improve rapport as the patient will feel able to speak more openly.

11-5   **Correct answer (a).**
Patients' intelligence can be estimated by an assessment of their vocabulary and fund of knowledge, which are good global markers of intelligence. Attention is usually assessed by determining how well the patient responds to questions and by formal tests such as 'serial sevens'. Memory and orientation are assessed using standard memory tests in the Mental State Examination. Abstract thinking is assessed by the patient's interpretation of a proverb, and judgment by asking how the patient would behave in a certain situation.

11-6   **Correct answers (b), (c).**
Questions about suicidal thoughts need to be direct; for example, 'Have you thought about killing yourself?'. Depressed patients are often suicidal and suicide is their major risk. It should always be assessed in depressed patients. Asking about it does not put the thought of suicide into a patient's head and does not increase the risk of a patient attempting suicide. It is pointless asking indirectly if a patient is contemplating suicide; it must always be done directly.

11-7   **Correct answer (c).**
Clouding of consciousness is a feature of delirium. Patients with schizophrenia or high anxiety may appear perplexed, but do not have clouding of consciousness. In dementia, there may be disturbances of memory and orientation, but not clouding of consciousness.

11-8   **Correct answers (d), (e).**
The Mental State Examination is a systematic recording of your observations of the patient. It also includes tests of cognitive function. The Mental State Examination is carried out throughout the course of the interview; it is not something that is done at the completion of the interview. It can be performed by any person trained in performing a Mental State Examination and is not only done by psychiatrists. It includes more than just tests of memory.

11-9   **1(c), 2(d), 3(e), 4(a), 5(b).**
   1(c). Depression is a common and normal emotion. It is only abnormal if it is persistent and interferes with normal functioning.

2(d). An obsession is a repetitive thought, known to be irrational, and resisted by the patient. It may lead to repetitive behaviour (compulsion) in patients with obsessive compulsive disorder.

3(e). A fear of a harmless object or animal is a common symptom. When mild it produces only minor inconvenience. Severe phobias can be very disruptive to normal life. The patient is usually aware that the fear is not logical.

4(a). Hallucinations can occur in any of the senses. In addition to occurring in psychotic illnesses, they can have an organic aetiology. For example, olfactory hallucinations occur typically as a result of sphenoid wing meningiomas.

5(b). Delusion is an irrational belief that no one else shares. Schizophrenia commonly results in delusional states. The patient for example may be convinced a radio transmitter has been secretly implanted in his brain to listen to his thoughts. These delusions are often technologically advanced.

Chapter 12
The Skin

12-1   Both statements are true.
Involvement of the neurovascular bundles or cutaneous nerves by certain skin diseases can cause anaesthesia. This is responsible for the deformities that occur in patients with leprosy.

12-2   Both statements are true.
There are a number of skin manifestations in systemic diseases. Some of these diseases may present with skin abnormalities in the first instance.

12-3   Correct answers (c), (d).
Sebaceous cysts can be felt to lie within the skin, but a number of other skin conditions can also present in this way. For example, secondary deposits may lie within the skin. A mass arising from the subcutaneous tissue may be fixed to the overlying skin particularly if it is a malignancy. If a mass appears to be within a muscle, contraction of the muscle will make the lump less mobile. Various nerve tumours will cause paraesthesiae in the distribution of the nerve if they are pressed. Lumps palpable over bone are not always tender; tenderness suggests infection.

12-4   Correct answers (a), (c), (e).
Cutaneous masses which contain fluid are fluctuant. This means that movement of fluid within the lump can be detected. Masses containing clear fluid will light up (transilluminate) when a torch is applied to them, but turbid or viscous fluids will not transilluminate. Masses resulting from inflammation usually produce redness, heat and tenderness in the overlying skin. An inflammatory mass will often have associated regional lymphadenopathy. Neurofibromas do not contain fluid.

12-5   Correct answers (a), (b), (d), (e).
There are many causes of itchiness of the skin. Cholestatic jaundice results in the deposition of bilirubin and other substances in the skin and subcutaneous tissues causing generalised itch. Pruritus is not uncommon in patients with lymphoma or chronic renal failure. Psychogenic causes are a common explanation of this problem. Addison's disease is not associated with pruritus.

12-6   Correct answers (c), (d), (e).
The lesions of secondary syphilis can occur on the palms and the soles but are not itchy.

Lichen planus lesions are usually itchy. Nummular eczema tends to be more diffuse. Psoriatic lesions are well demarcated and occur on extensor surfaces. Lesions of recent onset which are scattered over the trunk may be due to pityriasis rosea.

12-7   Correct answers (a), (b), (c), (d).
Blistering eruptions are common in viral infections such as herpes simplex and herpes zoster. Zoster lesions are confined in most cases to a single dermatome but do not spread far over the midline (they may occur slightly over the midline). Dermatitis herpetiformis causes very widespread and itchy lesions. Porphyria cutanea tarda is an important systemic disease. It is associated with blistering eruptions on the hands and may be related to hepatitis C infection. Deep blistering lesions may occasionally cause scarring, especially in patients with pemphigus vulgaris.

12-8   Both statements are true.
One of the rare dermatological emergencies is erythroderma where loss of skin results in massive fluid and electrolyte loss. This can be life-threatening.

12-9   First statement false, second statement true.
Pustular lesions contain dead neutrophils which may be there secondary to infection or inflammation.

12-10   Correct answers (b), (d), (e).
Erythema nodosum is characteristically found below the knee in the pretibial area. It is associated with inflammatory bowel disease (ulcerative colitis and Crohn's disease). It can also occur in patients with pulmonary tuberculosis. It is quite common in patients with sarcoidosis. It may occur from a drug reaction to penicillin or sulfonamides.

12-11   Correct answers (b), (c), (d), (e).
Hyperthyroidism rather than hypothyroidism is associated with increased sweating. It is also common in patients with acromegaly and of course fever. Episodes of hypoglycaemia can cause profound sweating. Some patients with autonomic dysfunction (e.g. related to long-standing diabetes mellitus) may sweat abnormally.

12-12   Both statements are true.
Skin ulcers which appear to be due to trauma or infection but do not heal can be the result of underlying malignancy and the diagnosis is best made by biopsy.

12-13   Correct answers (a), (d), (e).
Malignant melanoma occurs in fair skinned populations and the incidence is highest in the tropics. Overall skin exposure to sun seems important. Those who spend a lot of time in the sun are at increased risk. Solar keratoses indicate skin damage from sunlight and an increased risk of melanoma. The inherited condition dysplastic naevus syndrome puts people at very high risk of melanoma.

12-14   Correct answers (a), (b), (c), (d).
Dermatomyositis is an inflammatory muscle disease associated with characteristic lilac-covered flat-topped papules over the knuckles or a rash on the face. Patients with rheumatic fever may develop the characteristic erythema marginatum that spares the face. This is one of the major criteria for the diagnosis of rheumatic fever. Neurofibromatosis (Von Recklinghausen's disease) causes typical skin papules (subcutaneous neurofibromas) which look hard but feel soft and *café au lait* (cream-brown) spots on the skin. Infective endocarditis causes changes including splinter haemorrhages and, rarely, Osler's nodes. Although long-term steroid use can cause changes in skin fragility, recent short-term use is unlikely to cause any diagnostic changes.

Chapter 13
Infectious Diseases

13-1   Correct answers (d), (e).
Pyrexia of unknown origin is most often found to be due to the uncommon presentation of a common disease. Infective causes are more often diagnosed early. In most cases an explanation is found. Almost one-third of cases is associated with a malignancy. A significant proportion turn out to be the result of a connective tissue disease.

13-2   Correct answers (a), (b), (c), (d), (e).
Drug reactions are common causes of fever and rash. A new drug must always be considered a possible explanation of such symptoms. Syphilis can run a subacute course and may be associated with prolonged fever and skin changes. Viral infections including hepatitis B and C and HIV infection may lead to prolonged symptoms of this type. Connective tissue and inflammatory diseases should be considered in a patient with this presentation. Travel to tropical areas involves a risk of infection with parasites and exotic diseases such as typhoid.

13-3   Both statements are false.
Fungal infections can sometimes be a cause of prolonged fever and may be difficult to diagnose (e.g. blastomycosis, coccidioidomycosis, histoplasmosis).

13-4   Correct answers (a), (b), (c), (e).
The abdominal examination may often be rewarding in a patient with a difficult febrile illness. Occasionally, a tender abdominal mass may be found owing to the presence of an abscess. Inguinal lymphadenopathy may suggest the presence of lymphoma or chronic infection in the legs. Splenomegaly is a feature of many infective and malignant conditions. Enlarged para-aortic nodes are rarely palpable and do not occur in typhoid. A rectal mass may suggest a rectal abscess or malignancy.

13-5   Correct answers (a), (b), (d), (e).
Patients may appear well for many years after HIV infection and seroconversion. Wasting is very common with advanced disease. Treatment of atypical mycobacterial infection with clofazimine can cause deep pigmentation. Herpes zoster involving more than one dermatome is most common in the intermediate phase of the illness. The so-called seroconversion illness may occur a few weeks after exposure to the virus and cause a flu-like illness with a maculopapular rash. The lesions of Kaposi's sarcoma are commonly seen in patients with HIV/AIDS. They are raised purple lesions which are usually not tender.

13-6   Correct answers (a), (b), (c), (e).
A number of abnormalities may be present on the mucosal surfaces of the mouth and tongue. These include ulcers which may be aphthous or due to herpes simplex, the peculiar hairy leukoplakia and typical Kaposi's lesions. The presence of Kaposi's lesions in the mouth indicates a high probability that they will be present elsewhere in the gastrointestinal tract. Periodontal disease is also common because of reduced immunity. Macroglossia is not a feature of AIDS.

Final Quiz

R-1   Correct answers (a), (b), (c), (d).
The pain of pericarditis is usually pleuritic. Typically this is a sharp chest pain that is worse with deep breathing, because this causes the inflamed pericardial surfaces to rub

together. Exertional dyspnoea and cough (especially when the patient lies down) are symptoms of the cardiac failure which can accompany myocarditis. Atrial fibrillation may complicate myocarditis or pericarditis. Exertional chest tightness or pain is more suggestive of ischaemia.

R-2   Correct answers (a), (b), (c), (d), (e).
Oesophageal reflux may be a common cause of cough which may occur because of aspiration of small amounts of refluxed acid. A similar mechanism may cause hoarseness. Chronic blood loss from oesophageal ulceration can eventually lead to anaemia and lethargy. Recurrent reflux may cause oesophageal ulceration, and as this heals a stricture may develop. This can cause dysphagia.

R-3   Correct answers (a), (c), (d), (e).
Secondary infections are a late complication of HIV infection. Cytomegalovirus causes retinitis, oesophagitis, colitis and pneumonia. *Toxoplasma gondii* can produce encephalitis, brain abscess, chorioretinitis and myocarditis. Cryptosporidia and microsporidia can both cause diarrhoea, and no effective therapy is available. Echovirus infection is not a problem in AIDS patients.

R-4   Correct answers (a), (c), (d).
Active rheumatoid arthritis is associated with prolonged morning stiffness, the anaemia of chronic inflammatory disease and a larger number of involved joints. Fever and rheumatoid factor levels are not specific signs of activity.

R-5   Correct answers (a), (d).
The rather sudden onset of symptoms, especially of fever, is common in cases of bronchial pneumonia. Bronchial breath sounds are also present over the affected area from early in the illness.

R-6   Correct answer (c).
Unlike Crohn's disease, ulcerative colitis does not involve the full thickness of the colonic wall. For this reason fistulae do not usually occur. The commonest cause of chronic liver disease in ulcerative colitis is primary sclerosing cholangitis. Patients with long-standing colitis have an increased risk of colonic adenocarcinoma. Dehydration, as a result of diarrhoea, and toxic megacolon are acute complications.

R-7   Correct answers (a), (d), (e).
An asymmetrical and large goitre may cause tracheal displacement to either side. Removal of one lung will cause tracheal deviation towards that side. A tension pneumothorax will cause tracheal deviation away from the affected side while collapse of a lobe causes shift to the same side. Severe upper lobe fibrosis may pull the trachea towards the affected side.

R-8   Correct answers (a), (b), (d), (e).
Dry eyes are a characteristic symptom of Sjögren's syndrome. Interstitial lung disease, arthritis and parotid gland enlargement may complicate the disease. Parotid gland enlargement is usually, but not always, bilateral.

R-9   Correct answers (a), (c), (e).
Normochromic normocytic anaemia is a feature of chronic disease. It suggests inability of the bone marrow to produce enough red cells. After significant blood loss, haemodilution occurs and the blood film is at first normocytic. Then the reticulocyte count increases as more red cells are produced in response to the blood loss and the film may appear macrocytic. Iron deficiency prevents production of normal amounts of

haem, resulting in microcytosis. Microcytosis is also a feature of thalassaemia where it is a consequence of abnormal haem production.

R-10   Correct answers (a), (b), (c), (d).
Hypertrophic cardiomyopathy is characterised by abnormal thickening of the septum of the heart. Systolic anterior (not posterior) movement of the anterior mitral valve leaflet is a characteristic echocardiographic finding. This interference with mitral valve function by the hypertrophied septum can also result in mitral regurgitation. Patients have an increased risk of serious ventricular arrhythmias and therefore of sudden death. These patients also have a small risk of developing infective endocarditis.

R-11   Correct answers (a), (c), (d).
Patients with acute renal failure have usually had normal kidneys up to the time of the onset of failure. Chronic renal disease, however, usually results in a decrease in renal size over time. One exception is adult polycystic kidney disease, which is a cause of chronic renal failure in patients with palpable kidneys. Hyperkalaemia can be a result of acute or chronic renal disease. Nocturia suggests a loss of renal concentrating ability and may be an early symptom of renal disease; anaemia takes time to develop in these patients. The presence of red cell casts suggests acute glomerulonephritis and hence acute renal failure.

R-12   Correct answer (a).
Mitral valve prolapse is not associated with cardiac symptoms unless it has caused at least moderately severe mitral regurgitation. There may be no abnormal findings on auscultation (in this case the diagnosis will have been made on echocardiographic examination). Alternatively there may be a click or a late systolic murmur, or both. Review every five years is probably enough when the patient has only trivial or mild mitral regurgitation at the time of diagnosis. A small but significant proportion of these patients progress to develop mitral regurgitation severe enough to need valve repair or replacement.

R-13   Correct answer (a).
Spondylolisthesis refers to the slipping of the vertebral body, pedicles and superior articular facets in an anterior direction as a result of an injury (most often L5 on S1). Radiculopathy may or may not occur. Herniation of a disc is a major cause of chronic back (and leg) pain, but is rare in the thoracic spine. It may occur after a flexion injury but often no trauma is remembered by the patient.

R-14   Correct answer (a).
Memory loss for recent events is a common early symptom of dementia. Hypertension may be an association of multi-infarct dementia, but not of Alzheimer's disease. Deterioration of cognitive function is more gradual in Alzheimer's dementia than in multi-infarct dementia. Visuo-spatial tasks are not specifically affected in this disease. Personality changes occur but aggressive outbursts are not common.

R-15   Correct answers (a), (d), (e).
Hepatitis, cytomegalovirus (CMV) and HIV are well known risks following needlestick injury. CMV can be transmitted by contaminated blood transfusions.

R-16   Correct answers (a), (c), (d), (e).
Apart from lung cancer, these are all features of HIV infection or its complications.

R-17   Correct answers (a), (b), (c), (d), (e).
Elderly patients may become confused and incontinent as a result of any of a number of systemic insults. Any of the listed conditions may be responsible.

R-18   Correct answers (a), (e).
Rheumatoid arthritis is often but not always symmetrical. Early morning stiffness is a classical symptom. Rheumatoid nodules are an important sign. Iritis and ankylosing spondylitis can occur in seronegative arthritis but not in rheumatoid arthritis.

R-19   Correct answers (a), (c), (d), (e).
Migraine is usually unilateral but can affect both sides of the head. Women are more often affected than men. There is quite often a family history. Nausea is common. Migraine may be preceded by neurological symptoms in the territory of the artery involved. This is due to arterial spasm and resultant cerebral ischaemia. The headache is a result of the reflex arterial dilatation that follows.

R-20   Correct answers (a), (b), (c).
Fever is usually present in cases of septic arthritis. Possible sources include organisms from a skin infection and gonorrhoea.

R-21   Correct answers (b), (c).
The left middle cerebral artery supplies the left motor cortex. Damage here can cause right hemiparesis and failure of the eyes to deviate to the right. The eyes 'look at the lesion'. The motor area for speech may also be damaged and this causes dysphasia. The occipital lobes are not affected.

R-22   Correct answer (b)
Atrial fibrillation in a man of this age without other cardiac symptoms is likely to be self-limiting and not due to structural heart disease. Ischaemic heart disease is an unlikely but still possible cause. Alcohol can precipitate atrial fibrillation in some cases. Brucellosis is not an association. Thyrotoxicosis is an important cause.

R-23   Correct answers (a), (b), (c), (d).
Right ventricular failure is often secondary to chronic lung disease when this has caused chronic pulmonary hypertension. Recurrent deep venous thromboses that have caused significant pulmonary embolism can also cause pulmonary hypertension. The lung changes that occur in patients with sleep apnoea or severe obesity (or both) can have a similar outcome. In these conditions changes in lung mechanics caused by the increased work of breathing lead to a rise in pulmonary artery pressures. An unrepaired atrial septal defect may lead to pulmonary hypertension (and cyanotic congenital heart disease).

R-24   Correct answers (b), (e).
Most patients with infective endocarditis have fever as well as a significant valve lesion and associated murmur. Microscopic haematuria is also common and is probably due to immune-complex deposition in the glomeruli. Splenomegaly occurs in 30% of cases. The other phenomena are relatively uncommon and are not present in the majority of patients.

R-25   Correct answer (a).
The smoking of even 15 cigarettes a day increases the risk of a person's developing ischaemic heart disease, carcinoma of the lung and chronic airflow limitation. Small amounts of alcohol seem safe for both men and women. The consumption of some saturated fat is not a risk factor in itself but becomes so once a person's serum lipids are found to be elevated. Having a first-degree relative with ischaemic heart disease increases a person's own risk, but probably only if the affected relative was under 60 years of age. This is because ischaemic heart disease is common anyway in our society. Blood pressure varies considerably during a normal day. The systolic reading rises with exercise. A single recording at this level is of little significance.

R-26   Correct answers (b), (e).
Amenorrhoea is of course normal after the menopause, before the menarche and during pregnancy. Abdominal or indeed any irradiation of a pregnant woman may put the fetus at risk. Increases in the doses of therapeutic drugs are rarely required during pregnancy. However, the possible teratogenic effect of any drug must be considered before it is given to a pregnant woman or indeed before it is given to a woman of child-bearing age who may be pregnant without being aware of it. Ultrasound at diagnostic doses does not seem to pose any risk to the fetus. Menstruation is sensitive to systemic illnesses of many types. Amenorrhoea may occur with severe weight loss from any cause including anorexia nervosa.

R-27   Correct answer (a).
Pleural plaques are the most common result of asbestos exposure. Pulmonary fibrosis (**not** upper lobe) and mesothelioma (a malignant pleural tumour) are the other important sequelae.

R-28   Correct answers (a), (b), (d).
Interstitial lung disease and photosensitivity rashes are not features of Reiter's syndrome. Various patterns of arthritis may occur.

R-29   Correct answers (b), (c), (d), (e).
Prolonged early morning stiffness is a feature of rheumatoid arthritis. The other features listed are characteristic of osteoarthritis. The family history may be positive because of a genetic predisposition.

R-30   Correct answers (a), (d).
Life expectancy is definitely reduced for patients who develop dementia when they are compared with unaffected people of the same age. The mean period of survival, once dementia has been diagnosed, is eight years. The condition becomes more common with age, approaching 40% for those in their mid-80s. Alzheimer's disease is a more common cause of dementia than multi-infarct dementia, the next most common type. Dementia is not usually reversible. Rare exceptions include dementia secondary to vitamin B_{12} deficiency, hypothyroidism, drugs and chronic subdural haematoma.

R-31   Correct answers (a), (b), (e).
Viral causes of arthritis and rash include hepatitis B, rubella, HIV and arboviral diseases (e.g. Ross River virus in Australia). Serum sickness (e.g. as a result of drug hypersensitivity) causes fever, rash, arthralgia, lymphadenopathy and proteinuria. Gout is associated with arthritis but not rash, and measles with a rash but not with arthritis.

R-32   Correct answers (a), (b), (c), (d).
Gouty arthritis is more common in certain racial groups. Attacks can be precipitated by alcohol, are self-limiting (though extremely painful) and associated with gouty tophi. Fever is not common.

R-33   Correct answers (b), (c), (d), (e).
These are features of Reiter's syndrome. The organism that precipitates this syndrome cannot be cultured from synovial fluid.

R-34   Correct answers (a), (d), (e).
The palmomental and jaw jerk reflexes test frontal lobe dysfunction. The other reflexes involve the brainstem at some point in their reflex arc.

R-35   Correct answers (b), (d), (e).
Scabies is caused by infestation by the scabies mite which is not an insect. The hands and wrists are most often involved. The parasites are easily transmitted by both sexual and non-sexual contact.

R-36   Correct answers (a), (b), (c), (d).
Peripheral neuropathy is a very common complication of diabetes mellitus, and diabetes itself is common. Vasculitis of the vasa nervorum — the blood vessels which supply the nerves — can result in nerve damage which is scattered in different parts of the body. Motor nerves are more sensitive to demyelination than sensory ones. Demyelination causes severe loss of conduction velocity. Alcoholic neuropathy is probably more related to the vitamin B deficiency that occurs in those that are malnourished, than to a direct toxic effect.

R-37   Correct answers (a), (c), (d).
The lateral medullary syndrome consists of ipsilateral cerebellar signs and an ipsilateral Horner's syndrome with contralateral pain and temperature loss over the body. There may be ipsilateral pain and temperature loss on the face. It is one of the most dramatic syndromes in neurology.

R-38   Correct answers (a), (b), (c), (d).
The woman described clearly has acromegaly which should have been diagnosed years ago. Abdominal striae occur in Cushing's syndrome but not in acromegaly.

R-39   Correct answers (a), (b), (e).
Psoriasis is one of the most common chronic skin disorders. It is of unknown aetiology but is associated with increased epidermal cell turnover. It is not an immune complex disease and does not affect the small bowel (unlike dermatitis herpetiformis in coeliac disease). Five to ten percent of patients have arthritis.

R-40   Correct answer (e).
Subarachnoid haemorrhage causes meningism because of the irritating effect of blood in the subarachnoid space. Meningism does not occur in the other conditions.

R-41   Correct answers (b), (c), (d).
Parkinson's disease affects muscle control but does not directly reduce motor strength. Urinary incontinence is not a feature.

R-42   Correct answers (a), (b), (c), (d).
Squamous cell carcinomas (SCCs) are not pigmented. They are very common in patients on immunosuppression therapy following renal transplantation. These people must be very careful about sun exposure. Metastatic disease is rare but occurs occasionally in patients with advanced (neglected) tumours. Chronic skin ulcers may be complicated by SCCs. An ulcer which does not heal may be an SCC.

R-43   Correct answers (b), (c), (d), (e).
Malignant melanoma often metastasises once it has begun to penetrate the skin. These rather strange malignant lesions may disappear spontaneously even after they have become metastatic. They can appear *de novo* or in an existing mole.

R-44   Correct answers (a), (b).
Atopic eczema usually begins in childhood and is common when people also have other atopic conditions including rhinitis, asthma and conjunctivitis. It is not associated with psoriasis and is an allergic rather than an autoimmune disease.

R-45   Correct answer (b).
This patient has severe diabetic retinopathy. The new vessel formation is destructive and will cause gross interference with vision. It is now clear that tight control of blood sugar levels does reduce the risk of diabetic complications, including retinopathy. This patient's visual loss will not be correctable with spectacles since it is not a refractive problem. Changes of this sort suggest that the patient has been diabetic for at least some years.

R-46   Correct answers (b), (c), (d).
Diabetes insipidus (failure of secretion of antidiuretic hormone) is not associated with a change in facial appearance. Patients with mitral stenosis may have a characteristic malar flush, but this is common only in severe mitral stenosis.

R-47   Correct answer (b).
Many pathological murmurs are not associated with symptoms until cardiac decompensation has occurred. Innocent murmurs are usually soft and may be difficult to hear. Diastolic murmurs are pathological unless part of a venous hum (and in this case both systolic and diastolic components are long). The presence of a thrill strongly suggests that a murmur is pathological. Fixed splitting of the second heart sound is a sign of an atrial septal defect.

R-48   Correct answer (a).
This patient has obviously had a spontaneous pneumothorax. There may be no signs at all or merely a reduction in breath sounds over the affected lobe.

R-49   Both answers are false.
Breath sound are normally bronchial in character over the main bronchi, hence the name.

R-50   Correct answers (a), (b), (d).
Generalised pruritus can be due to systemic disease. However, adrenal failure and acromegaly do not cause pruritus.

R-51   Correct answers (a), (b), (e).
Exposure to vibrating machines of various sorts and to the poison, vinyl chloride, can lead to Raynaud's phenomenon. It is also common in some connective tissue diseases but not in diabetes or infective endocarditis.

You will have to learn many tedious things, . . . which you will forget the moment you have passed your final examination, but . . . it is better to have learned and lost than never to have learned at all.

W Somerset Maugham
(1874–1965)